un*healthy
Living Well.
ANONYMOUS

D1114581

unhealthy ANONYMOUS

Living Well.

EXPOSING THE GREATEST THREAT TO YOUR

Health & Happiness

Dr. Pete Sulack

DESTINY IMAGE® PUBLISHERS, INC.

P.O. Box 310, Shippensburg, PA 17257-0310

"Promoting Inspired Lives."

This book and all other Destiny Image and Destiny Image Fiction books are available at Christian bookstores and distributors worldwide.

Cover design by: Prodigy Pixel

Manuscript assistance by Dr. Dori Anne Abbott and Rick Killian

For more information on foreign distributors, call 717-532-3040.

Reach us on the Internet: www.destinyimage.com.

ISBN 13 TP: 978-0-7684-0688-7

ISBN 13 eBook: 978-0-7684-0689-4

For Worldwide Distribution, Printed in the U.S.A.

2 3 4 5 6 7 8 / 19 18 17 16 15

"If you know the enemy and know yourself, you need not fear the result of a hundred battles. If you know yourself but not the enemy, for every victory gained you will also suffer a defeat. If you know neither the enemy nor yourself, you will succumb in every battle."

—SUN TZU

Contents

We're in a Fight for Our Lives

They have come from far and wide over the last decade—people with no hope. Individuals who have been to specialist after specialist, but who still remain confused and hopeless about the answer to the question, "What happened to my health, and how can I get it back?" We've learned how to extend the length of human life, but what good is it if the quality of that life is lousy?

Do you feel lousy? Are you too tired to do all the things you dreamed of doing? Do you take multiple medications every day? Do you spend a lot of time managing your symptoms? If so, you are not alone, and I would say to you, "There is hope!" If you are one of those people who is searching for answers to your health problems and has put up with dehumanizing surgeries, has been put on medications that have worse side effects than the original conditions, this book is for you! I humbly say to you—*this is it!* Not the next fad diet or medical craze. Simply, these are the steps out of the mess you are in—the 12 steps to silencing the silent killer: Stress!

We all talk about stress; we all know it is harmful to our health; but we don't ever really address the stressors in our lives. We don't treat the stress systemically—at its source. We treat the symptoms of stress like high blood pressure, weight gain, fatigue, brain fog, sexual dysfunction, or heart disease; but we don't really treat the stress! We have an enemy in the camp whose face is familiar, whose habits are obvious—an enemy with whom we sleep and eat. If we don't neutralize this enemy, we will lose the battle for health and happiness. These 12 seeds or stepping stones will do that. They are the necessary steps to transform your life and health—to help you recapture what you thought was gone forever!

If the captain of the Titanic had realized the importance of slowing down and had recognized the danger of that iceberg in the North Atlantic, history would have turned out differently! So if you are having a health crisis, or if you are headed toward that inevitable iceberg, take heart! You are about to change your own history! Personally, I would rather be at death's door and be moving in the right direction than to assume that every-thing is fine and be moving in the wrong direction. Together we will right the ship of your life and get you moving in the right direction.

Will it be new? Absolutely! Will it be uncomfortable and chal-lenging? Sometimes. A lot of what I will share in this book will be a new perspective or paradigm of health. Once you begin to see the need to "slow down," and realize the danger of the "icebergs" ahead of you, change will come naturally, and you will regain a vibrancy, youthfulness, and joy you never thought possible! Until the enemy of stress is exposed, we will *never* get the victory! So, let's get started!

ONE WOMAN'S STORY

For the great enemy of truth is very often not the lie—deliberate, contrived, and dishonest—but the myth—persistent, persuasive, and unrealistic. Too often we hold fast to the clichés of our forebears. We subject all facts to a prefabricated set of interpretations. We enjoy the comfort of opinion without the discomfort of thought. —JOHN F. KENNEDY

Deanna had no idea what to do. She had been suffering for nearly 30 years. She had been to numerous doctors, and desperately needed some real answers. Almost 20 years ago she'd had two radical surgeries to remove her colon as a treatment for the ulcerative colitis she had suffered with for almost a decade. While this seemed to help, she still wondered why none of the "experts" had really ever understood her condition or knew how to manage it long term. Surgery had seemed a last resort; and even after she'd had that surgery, she found herself constantly returning to the doctor to manage the symptoms that continued to plague her.

Sometime after surgery, she was diagnosed with Hashimoto's Thyroiditis, another autoimmune disease. This caused her tremendous anxiety because she knew that most autoimmune issues can eventually lead to more serious health conditions and even death. It was one of the reasons she had agreed to have her colon surgically removed in the first place, and now it seemed as if she were right back where she had started. The doctors gave her prescriptions to manage her Hashimoto's. Feeling some relief from her symptoms, she assumed she had finally found her path to recovery through surgery, medication, and regular checkups.

Despite her medications and constant checkups, about three years ago she began to experience a new series of bizarre symptoms—nine months of severe hives, frightful chemical sensitivities requiring her to carry an EpiPen at all times, constant heart palpitations, burning feet, restless legs, insomnia, a benign tumor on her parathyroid (which she had to have surgically removed), vision disturbances, bowel troubles (even though she had no colon), hormonal havoc, distressing fatigue, raging anxiety, and uncontrollable weight loss. If all of that wasn't bad enough, depression hovered over her constantly, saturating her mind with dark thoughts and emotions. She wasn't sure what to do. This was no kind of life.

Deanna's health issues affected every part of her existence. She was forced to leave the job she loved as a middle school teacher. Over the next two years, she saw 16 different doctors who prescribed a number of different dangerous medications—enough to stagger the imagination. Despite these, she saw no real change in her symptoms, and her health concerns grew steadily worse.

Deanna wasn't a quitter! She knew she hadn't been brought into this world to suffer without reason. She knew that for every problem there is a solution. She prayed for guidance, and she had faith that she would receive that guidance. She began to study how the body works, and spent hours on the Internet trying to understand her ailments and the possible diseases causing them. She continued to pray and meditate daily over the information she found, looking for what she should do next. As Deanna continued to look for answers, she found out about our clinic and made an appointment for a consultation.

When she shared her history with me, I explained our philosophy that the body is designed to heal itself, but it needs to be restored to proper function in order to do so. We partnered with Deanna in her quest to heal her body, and then we transitioned her into learning how to keep her body healthy in the future. She was delighted that as she incorporated the changes we suggested, she began to get better! That was about three years ago. Recently Deanna wrote to us:

> Today I have *no* anxiety, *no* hives, *no* restless legs, *no* heart palpitations, and *no* depression! Every symptom—*gone!* I have more than completely recovered! ...I lived decades without knowing how to respect this body, but *no more!*
>
> ...I am so grateful for the compassion and hope I found through meeting Dr. Pete and the staff. It was in their office that I began to truly learn about the real power of foods—the good stuff and the bad stuff. The Internet became a powerful resource as I researched ferociously. I have exited the halls of the conventional approach, and am taking personal responsibility for the answers I need!
>
> Today, I experience so much daily joy! I take no medications! ...I thank God for always providing exactly what we need!

THE SAME CAN HAPPEN TO YOU!

You may not be suffering as significantly as Deanna was, but the answers she found are the same for anyone who wants to live a healthier, happier life. Our bodies are perhaps the most incredible creations in the universe! Our internal systems have been masterfully designed to propel toward health, fight disease, and be strong when we maintain them in a state of balance or *homeostasis*. Homeostasis is the state of balance that all living beings return to when their systems are operating in a healthy way. It is the exact opposite of stress. The best part is that finding your homeostasis, living in balance, and achieving this ideal state is entirely under your control!

We hear about stress all the time in the media, but no one is really addressing it at its source. Citizens of developed countries have more sickness, more disease, and are more overweight than any human beings in recorded history. We face more stressors, more toxins, and are getting less nutrition from our food than any generation that has gone before us. The medical model of attacking sickness and disease has focused solely on making the acutely sick or injured well. It has yet to come up with a solution to the epidemic of chronic disease caused by our modern lifestyles and toxic, harmful environments. Certainly medical practitioners can save a life in the midst of a heart attack and prescribe medications designed to alleviate symptoms, but sending those patients right back to the same suicidal lifestyle habits is a guarantee of future failure.

Now I'm not trying to knock doctors—they are some of the most caring people on the planet; but over the last century or so, the medical paradigm from which they have operated has failed us miserably! While modern medicine can help people in the midst of crises, true cures for the chronic illnesses of today are elusive. No matter how much money is thrown at these problems, there are still no real, satisfying answers.

Cardiovascular disease; cancer; type 2 diabetes; autoimmune diseases like Multiple Sclerosis, Parkinson's, and Crohn's disease; Alzheimer's dementia; and other chronic ailments that affect roughly 80 percent of our population are not getting better; they are increasing exponentially! This is because the modern medical paradigm is reductionist by nature. It focuses on fixing what is broken in one body system while paying little attention to the wisdom of the body and the interaction of the body as a whole. Its best attempt at prevention is prescribing medications to address symptoms and risk factors. However, it is not focused on building and strengthening people so that they can endure the rigors of this life. Nor is it focused on building systems that won't break in the first place. They know how to address many of *the symptoms* of diseases with pharmaceuticals or surgery, but not how to heal the systems so that the body can combat disease on its own. Not only that, but the tools they use for fixing chronic illness often come with unpleasant or dangerous side effects that rival the diseases themselves. Why? Because pharmaceuticals developed in the last few centuries suppress symptoms, but they don't give our bodies the building blocks needed to create health. What will give us those building blocks?

- Detoxifying the body from inside and outside.

- Caging the tiger of stress that is taxing our bodies to the breaking point.

- Supplying our bodies with the nutrition and mobility they need so that our systems can function at peak efficiency, repair what is out of sync, and get us back to living healthier, happier lives.

Thousands of years ago, Hippocrates, the great physician, said, "Let food be thy medicine." He knew that the natural healing force within each of us—the body's innate intelligence—is the greatest force for getting well. It is time to get back to the wisdom of the ages that so many have forgotten.

In an effort to help people regain their health and vibrancy, we started Unhealthy Anonymous. This community allows us to teach and spread the insights we've gained over the years to any groups around the world that want the information. We don't claim to have all the answers. In fact, when I started my practice, I was stuck in the same paradigm as most of our culture. I believed many of the same myths that have been held sacred for decades:

- that eating fat causes the body to get fat

- that red meat causes heart disease

- that I should eat every couple of hours to maintain my blood sugar

- that all calories are equal

- that dieting is a simple formula of eating less and exercising more

- that breakfast is the most important meal of the day

- that grains should occupy the biggest portion of our dietary intake

However, with the insight of thousands of clinical observations and the help of several of my colleagues who are leaders in the field of health and nutrition, I have changed my entire perspective. As a result of this wisdom, we now teach these insights to anyone who seeks the foundation of true health. The truths we share in this book are revolutionary, life enhancing—and best of all, simple to understand and incorporate.

I know how confusing information about health and nutrition can be. It seems like everyone has a different idea. As I write this, four of the top ten best sellers for "Advice and Miscellaneous" are books focused on diet and health—and none of them agree as to what really works best for people. Some argue against grains and gluten, some against dairy and/or animal products, others urge us to eat like cavemen or nomads, and still others suggest we should never eat anything that can't be grown in a garden or an orchard.

On the surface, all of this information can seem contradictory and be quite confusing. However, as you delve into what is being taught as the new psychology of nutrition, you will realize that it sounds a lot like what ancient cultures prescribed for us to eat thousands of years ago. Each of us is powerfully unique, but the quest to create bodies that can adapt to and recover from stress rests on the unchanging principles of human design. This ability of the body to return again and again to a place of homeostasis or rest is the cornerstone of true health. If we get the cornerstone right, the rest of the building will stand.

My desire in writing this book and creating Unhealthy Anonymous is to partner with you and your loved ones—to help you get healthy and stay healthy by giving you the best information available. It's my goal to start a conversation that will make our nation healthier, one struggling person at a time.

As an added bonus for purchasing this book, you can go to our website, www.unhealthyanonymous.com to get our 21-day Reboot program for absolutely no cost. One thing our members have noticed is that when they follow the 21-day Reboot, they crave healthier and more wholesome foods rather than the stuff that is causing them to gain weight and setting them up for long-term disease. When you register for this program on our website, you will find shopping lists, recipes, and complete weekly meal plans to get you started on a healthier lifestyle. The hope is, by the end of those three weeks, you will be practiced enough in meal planning and have your appetite healed enough that you will get a vision and desire for a lifetime of proper nutrition and health.

My hope is that this book will become a great resource for you as you seek to create and live a more abundant life. You may ask, "How can a book keep up with the latest information that is out there?" The truth is, it really can't. Because of that, we have started an online community of people who desire the same as you – a happier and healthier life. By linking to www .unhealthyanonymous.com, you can stay up to date, inspired, motivated, and connected to others who have the same goals as you do of living healthier, happier lives.

What we've learned over the years in our practice and in the extensive charitable work we do around the world is that *changing the world* always starts with changing *your* world first. Until you can take the first small steps to getting control of your health, you cannot take the bigger steps of creating a life you love and sharing that life with the world at large. We want to see you take these initial steps—all 12 of them—in order to accomplish what you were put on the earth to do! I hear people all the time saying, *I'm too tired for that*, or, *if I had more energy, I would do this or that*. God wants us to live abundantly! And this includes having enough energy to accomplish our work in the world—whatever that may be. We want to empower and revitalize you so you can do just that. This a huge part of why we created Unhealthy Anonymous, and why we are building it through communities of like-minded people seeking to steward their bodies, their talents, and the other resources they have been given. I will give you 12 seeds to plant, and this community of like-minded individuals will be the soil that will allow the seeds (steps) to grow (germinate) into a mighty harvest of health and happiness! So, are you ready to get started?

Be blessed!

DR. PETE

Step One

Identify

People are fed by the food industry,
which pays no attention to health,
and are treated by the health industry,
which pays no attention to food.
—WENDELL BERRY

A s with any problem, the first step is to identify that there indeed is a problem. Once you realize this, then you can determine what that problem is and begin searching for strategies that will solve it. Many of us recognize that we would like to be thinner, have more energy, and live happier, healthier lives. Although we realize this, it often feels like the distance between where we are and where we want to be is a chasm wider than the Grand Canyon! Lord knows we've tried to eat healthier, started ambitious exercise programs, signed up for weight-loss plans, and bought volumes of new cookbooks. Time and again we lose momentum and then quit within a matter of weeks, if not days.

The arduous endeavor of getting from point A—where we are now—to where we would like to be at a very distant point Z— the trim, healthy, flexible, energetic, happy person we believe we should be—is just too great and too difficult to navigate.

If that even remotely describes you, I have good news for you: Change is not as hard as you think.

You have probably heard promises like this before. *So what, you may be asking, makes Unhealthy Anonymous different?* Well, first of all, thousands of other folks just like you have partnered with us to change their lives; and those changes have come to them. They are changes that they know they can live with for the rest of their lives. And the fact that they feel so much better and have more energy and a fresh vision for what is possible assures them that they will stay on track!

Second, Unhealthy Anonymous is more than a diet or exercise program. It's different because its main emphasis is on neutralizing the stress that is destroying your health, and creating a community of people working together towards the same health goals. As Dr. Mark Hyman wrote in his best-selling book, *The Blood Sugar Solution 10-Day Detox Diet,*

> When it comes to weight loss, studies show that social threads have a bigger impact than genetics. When people join together to lose weight and get healthy, not only is it more effective, it's also more fun! Losing weight is a team sport.[1]

And how does he know? Dr. Hyman was one of the advising physicians for The Daniel Plan conducted at Pastor Rick Warren's Saddleback Church in Orange County, California. During the first week, 15,000 participants signed up for the program, and in the first year those people lost an estimated 250,000 pounds! But that wasn't the most startling discovery. What was? According to Dr. Hyman, "The research indicated that *those who did the plan together lost twice as much weight as those who did it alone.*"[2] It's best to team up if you want to get healthy and stay healthy.

Third, Unhealthy Anonymous is about finding out what works best for *you*. Sure, there are some overarching principles that apply to the vast majority of us—sugar is a toxin; wheat, rye, and barley glutens cannot be digested so they encourage inflammation; good fats will help curb your appetite; etc.—but each of us is unique in body, soul, spirit, and purpose. One person's practice will not necessarily work for another in the same way. However, when we are working together, there is knowledge and insight available to us that would not be there otherwise. On your own, you may struggle to solve a particular challenge, but as a team, you will have access to the myriad of ideas that have worked for others.

WAKE-UP CALL

Over the past 20 years, there has been a dramatic increase in obesity of North Americans. More than one-third of U.S. adults (35.7 percent or 78.6 million) and approximately 17 percent (or 12.5 million) of children and adolescents aged 2–19 years are obese.[3]

We are bringing communities together with Unhealthy Anonymous—determining what works best for ourselves and our families, while sharing our successes and what we have learned with each other. We will encourage one another, pool our research so each person doesn't have to read every new book on transforming health, and work together to find the most fulfilling ways to create lives that we love. All of this comes back to step one: identifying our real problem.

#1) IDENTIFY THE ENEMY

If you purchased this book or received it when you showed up for your first Unhealthy Anonymous meeting, you have probably already come to the awareness that there are some health issues in your life, or the lives of your loved ones, that you want to solve. You may have a situation like Deanna, whose story you read in the introduction. Perhaps you have a chronic condition that you want to see improve. You may be concerned about your family history of cancer or heart disease. You may want to lose weight, feel better, and have more energy. Every person picking up this book will have a different reason for doing so, and each and every reason is valid.

No matter your reason for picking up this book, I have good news for you. Regardless of your health goals or challenges, the foundation for alleviating, healing, or in many cases preventing health challenges begins with facilitating your body's natural inborn ability to adapt to and recover from stress.

We all have stress—it's inescapable. In fact, stress is really what makes life challenging and fulfilling. It is often in overcoming stressful challenges that we find life's deeper meaning. At the same time, however, stress must be properly managed or it will become destructive. Giving our bodies what they need to cope with and recover from stress begins with changing our lifestyle choices.

These are choices like the way we eat, how much we exercise, how much time we allow for recovery, and how we manage our reactions to life's adversities. It has to do with adding the right foods and activities first, then slowly eliminating the foods and practices that are detrimental to your overall health.

Don't be alarmed about changing what you eat. I want you to know that the Unhealthy Anonymous plan is not about radically transforming your diet from day one, nor is it about starving yourself or adding a crushing amount of exercise. The focus of our program is to get you moving in a positive direction. It's all about building momentum and victory over time. When you start getting proper nutrition from what you eat, you will restore your body's innate ability to crave the foods that it needs the most. By modifying what you eat, you actually begin to change what you *want* to eat. You begin to crave more nutritious foods, not the stuff that is slowly killing you. As you get more nutrition, your body will get healthier, your hormones will balance, and your body will start to heal itself. You don't have to starve yourself. Instead, you will find that you are well fed, have great energy and feel much better. This ensures that you will stay with the program for better reasons than just weight loss. We don't want you to lose weight to get healthy; instead, we want you to get healthy and stay healthy. Then you will shed the weight.

While this is a simple plan, it doesn't necessarily mean it's a walk in the park. Changing your lifestyle doesn't happen overnight, and the habits you have formed—getting the same latte and pastry for breakfast every day, snacking endlessly while watching TV, being sedentary, ordering a diet Coke with every meal—will take some time and concerted effort to change. It takes real determination and focus to learn new habits, and the Unhealthy Anonymous program is designed to stack the deck in your favor.

Our program is designed to be more about joy and empowerment than it is about sacrifice and struggle.

For now, however, we simply want to acknowledge that the first step in solving most of our health issues begins with identifying the true enemy. In any battle, you can't be successful if you don't know who or what the enemy really is. That gives us a simple, common place to start, and allows us to move on to developing a clear vision of where we are headed.

 MYTH VS. FACT

Myth:
"I feel healthy, so I am healthy."

Fact:
Imagine, if you will, a battlefield. Both sides have been fighting for weeks with heavy casualties. On the one side, an army serving a totalitarian dictator who seeks world domination. On the other side, a group of freedom fighters—locals who don't want to see their land taken over by a madman. The commanding officer of the freedom fighters is burdened with the battle. No matter what approach he takes with his men, he is met with resistance at every turn. It's as if the enemy knows his every move. But how can they? Some days he doesn't plan his move until the last minute before he engages the enemy. He trusts a few good men; career men who would give their lives for him at a moment's notice. What he doesn't know is that one of those men is a traitor. He spies on the freedom fighters, and reports to the enemy on a regular basis. As long as the commander doesn't recognize this fact, and identify him as the enemy, the freedom fighters will continue to lose men until they

have to retreat or surrender. The end is already spelled out. The war is already lost. No matter how well they plan, how prepared they are, how hard they fight, or how ferociously they stick to their war plan, until that spy is identified and neutralized, they will continue to lose.

Every day people are diagnosed with dental disease (cavities), heart disease (high blood pressure/cholesterol), and all types of cancer (breast, colon, prostate) and don't even feel a single pain, lump, sensitivity or symptom. Many suffer heart attacks, cancer, strokes, and other "sudden" illnesses when they feel perfectly healthy—some even immediately after seemingly good checkups with their doctors.

How you feel doesn't matter as much as what is really happening inside your body. Not only that, but most of us don't really feel as healthy as we think we do—we have just gotten used to masking fatigue with caffeine, aches with medications, and chalking up symptoms to our age rather than what is really causing them.

Until we identify that stress is the enemy in our own camp, then it won't matter how much we try to eat right, or exercise, or take vitamins. Ultimately we will lose the battle to get healthy and stay healthy because we aren't fighting the right enemy. We are just shadow boxing.

You want to feel really healthy? Then realize and act on the fact that stress is your biggest enemy in the fight for health! You will be surprised how fit, strong, and healthy you can be even into your 80s and 90s if you just identify and neutralize the stressors on your body, and give it what it needs to begin once again to adapt to and recover from those stressors.

#2) IDENTIFY YOUR VISION

I use the word *vision* rather than *goals* because a vision is much more holistic than a list of individual objectives. As far as goals go, we tend to look for numerical changes such as lowering our blood pressure, LDL cholesterol counts, or losing X number of pounds. A vision, however, includes the motives behind why you set those goals, as well as how they work into your lifestyle. It includes the strategies and character with which you want to achieve those goals, as well as a practical understanding of the challenges you will face along the way and the realistic recognition of the amount of work necessary to see your vision become a reality.

There is a Jewish proverb that says: "*Where there is no vision, the people perish.*" However, when you look at the original Hebrew for this phrase, it doesn't really say, "*the people perish,*" but rather "*the people are unrestrained*" or "*cast off restraint.*" Why are people undisciplined in the pursuit of their goals? It's not because there's anything wrong with them, and it's not because there's anything wrong with their goals. It's because they don't have a compelling vision that motivates them to stick to their plan. If we don't have self-control, the problem isn't that we are weak-willed—the problem is we lack vision.

People can go to the other extreme as well. They focus in so tightly on their goals that they forget why they are trying to achieve them in the first place. They make unnecessary trade-offs and compromises to achieve the numbers, but they lose on other fronts like relationships or quality of life. So, for instance, people will radically change their lifestyles or starve themselves to get to their ideal weight, but they forget that the real point was to live a healthier and happier lifestyle that they can maintain. Not only do they compromise their health getting to their goals, but after they reach them, they find they can't maintain the lower weight without continuing to starve and work out at a feverish pace. They got what they wanted, but they lost the "Why?" behind it.

We don't attain what we causally set out to accomplish—we're just not designed that way. We obtain what we envision passionately. When we spend time adding to and developing a vision for the life we want, that vision becomes a powerful force, pulling us toward its fulfillment. What we visualize in our mind's eye changes us. Our habits change. Our thinking changes. Our willpower aligns with our vision, and our expectations become more magnetic. This is why professional athletes use visualization techniques as well as disciplined practice to hone their skills. Our minds don't differentiate between what we have done in our imaginations and what we practice in reality. When we see ourselves doing things the right way over and over and over again, it affects how we perform.

 MYTH VS. FACT

Myth:
Having fast-food French fries now and again never hurt anyone.

Truth:
High temperature frying, especially of potatoes, creates the chemical *acrylamide*. The fats used to fry fast food also stay in the body for many days causing a decrease in nerve transmission, increased hyperactivity, decreased immunity, and an increased risk for diabetes, cancer, and heart disease.

The point of having a vision is to focus on the results rather than on the pain of achieving those results. When we focus on the pain, we tend to give up; when we focus on the rewards, we keep working until we achieve them. It can be as simple as focusing on what you will feel like after you work out rather than how much you don't want to get out of bed. Realizing how much better you will feel sitting down to a healthy, home-cooked meal with your family rather than driving out to get fast food and eating it in the car. The key is to pull future rewards into your present state of mind and focus on the benefits rather than on the obstacles.

The more we develop and contemplate our vision, the more it becomes part of who we are. It doesn't take long for what we reflect on in our minds to become the reflection we see in the mirror! An unclear or ambivalent picture of how you want to look won't be enough to propel you towards achieving your ultimate goals. You need a detailed vision that you nurture, develop, and meditate on every day.

#3) IDENTIFY YOUR PLAN

Another crucial component of creating a healthier, happier life is proper planning. Most of us fall into eating at fast-food restaurants and buying convenience foods in the supermarket not because we are weak or don't have time to do better. Most of the time we drop the ball because we fail to have a better plan. When you make decisions while you are tired or stressed, the default setting is to do what you've always done. However, if you have a written plan, the easiest thing to do becomes to follow your plan!

Planning today is easier than it has ever been. There are apps for your smart phone that allow you to synchronize shopping lists between family members. You can set alarm reminders for preparing food ahead of time so you are ready to cook dinner at the same time every night. There are websites galore with health tips, recipes, downloadable meal plans and shopping lists, as well as video exercise programs. There are even YouTube videos that show you everything from how to set up your kitchen to walking you step by step through meal preparation. It has never been easier to learn about how to create a healthier, happier life and then planning and incorporating that plan into your weekly routine.

IT'S NOT ENTIRELY YOUR FAULT

In the last 40 years, the world has become increasingly more industrialized, and stress is at an all-time high. Our society looks nothing like it did just a generation ago. Over the last two decades, the number of unhealthy, diseased, overweight, and obese North Americans has skyrocketed. People have more chronic health issues than ever before, and are on more medications than ever before. This isn't because you have bad genes or are just getting older. This isn't an epidemic that has happened because of a change in climate, or because our generation is lazier than any before. If I were going to identify one factor, it wouldn't be that we watch more TV, play more video games, or surf the Internet more than we ever have before. The real issue is that our bodies are stressed. We have more stress than we have ever had in recorded human history. When we refer to stress at this point, I mean that stress is anything that puts an undue burden on the body. Some stress is good, but chronic stress with no relief is devastating to your health.

One of the many reasons that we are stressed is that our food supply has changed so dramatically. We put certain things into our bodies that should never have been called food. Just because something gives energy (calories) doesn't mean that it is food. If man created it, or it is filled with preservatives, or sits on the shelf for-ever, it has more than likely been altered in harmful ways. Look at margarine; it's not a real food. It is a combination of artifi-cial chemicals that give a certain taste. We put it in our mouths, but it is not a naturally occurring substance. Now we can taste strawberries in a syrup that has no strawberries in it. It is just a fabricated chemical designed to taste like a strawberry. Even at times when we think we are making a healthy food choice like vegetables, we learn that the process of industrial farming has stripped those foods of value and they now create more harm than good. America's topsoil is depleted, and the very DNA of food has been altered for reasons of economic efficiency and convenience. These factors of modern life all put complicated chemical stress on our bodies.

In order for topsoil to stay fertile, it must be cared for with good conservation practices. Unfortunately that is not happen-ing today. In order for plants to thrive, the soil in which they are grown must contain vast amounts of naturally occurring potassium, nitrogen, and phosphorous, as well as hundreds of trace minerals. Soil conservation is a set of strategies that pre-vent erosion or chemical alteration from overuse, acidification, salinization, or contamination. Strategies like crop rotation and planting cover crops and windbreaks are necessary steps to pro-tect our topsoil and help it to retain its integrity. The current use of glycophosphate (also known as "Roundup") in standard farming practices has poisoned our food supply. Even those who choose fruits and vegetables over junk food find their bodies assaulted by toxins that cause chronic stress, genetic mutations, and cell death. The company Monsanto, with their push for acceptance of these chemicals and acceptance of genetically modified foods, will someday be responsible for more human deaths than any totalitarian dictator in history![4]

The standard American diet today is higher in sugars, bad fats, bad carbohydrates, sodium, and other nutritionally bankrupt and downright harmful ingredients than ever before. We are paying the price for not getting enough of the right things in our food and getting too much of the wrong things. We are eating more than ever before, while our bodies think they are starving. Simply put, our food supply lacks the proper nutrition. As a result, we are constantly storing fat because our bodies are tricked into thinking that because nutrients are scarce, food must be scarce. We are coming to a time when being overweight is going to be a greater world issue than poverty and hunger. We are very close to seeing more people on earth dying from the associated diseases and conditions of obesity than from being underweight or starving.[5]

The processed foods that line grocery store shelves today have been carefully engineered to be as addictive as cigarettes or drugs. This is especially true of those that have added sugar, salt, fats, carbohydrates, or some diabolical combination of the four. Many of these processed foods—even ones that advertise themselves as "healthy," "whole," "gluten-free," and "organic"—don't have nearly the nutritional value that foods grown or raised in the right environment do. We need to recognize that much of what we eat out of habit is not because we lack willpower or self-control, but because those foods have been deliberately designed to be addictive. At the same time they have so little nutrition in them that they leave us hungrier than we were before we ate them. Then, to feel satisfied we binge— reaching for foods that please the palate, but stress our internal systems because they have so little of what our bodies really need.

✳ WAKE-UP CALL

Obesity-related conditions like heart disease, stroke, type 2 diabetes, and certain types of cancer are some of the leading causes of *preventable* death in our country today.

Despite such complications, the answer is relatively simple: As individual families and as a culture, we need to get back to eating real foods. When you eat real foods in the right combinations, something amazing happens—you feel full much sooner, and your appetite remains satisfied much longer. Your body is getting the fiber and nutrients that it needs. Your hunger hormones balance, and your appetite switches off. If your systems have been out of whack for a long time, this balance will take time to correct.

I want to warn you up front that you will be in for a bit of a fight, especially in the first few days. Food addiction is a real thing. When you eat gluten (wheat protein), casein (milk protein), and sugar, your brain is flooded with chemicals that make you feel calm and content. As you begin to remove those substances from your diet, you may feel some anxiety, or other physical effects. Hang in there. With each passing day your body will adjust, and your cravings will diminish. You will find that it takes about seven to ten days to do most of the work of recalibrating your appetite. This will vary depending on what your eating habits were like before beginning.

At the same time, by the end of the 21-day Reboot you will be surprised at how much your eating habits and appetites will have changed. You'll know something is different when you look forward to a hardy spinach salad with avocado, roasted pine nuts, wild-caught salmon, and a little feta cheese rather than a super-sized burger, fries, and a shake! And, oh boy, when that starts to happen, things start to get exciting!

NOTES

1.   Mark Hyman, MD, *The Blood Sugar Solution 10-Day Detox Diet: Activate Your Body's Natural Ability to Burn Fat and Lose Weight Fast* (New York: Little, Brown and Company, 2014), 11.

2.   Ibid., 69 [the italics are from the original].

3.   Overweight and Obesity," *Center for Disease Control and Prevention* website, http://www.cdc.gov/obesity/data/facts.html (accessed: August 13, 2014).

4.   A recent Harris poll put Monsanto as the third most hated corporation in the world—ranking only above BP and Bank of America. http://www.globalresearch.ca/monsantos-gamble -biotech-lobby-pushes-genetically-modified-gm-food-into -europe/5400307. For poll info: http://www.businessweek. com/articles/2014-07-03/gmo-factory-monsantos-high -tech-plans-to-feed-the-world.

5.   *Obesity: Preventing and Managing the Global Epidemic* (Geneva: World Health Organization, 2000), Introduction.

Step Two

Connect

Remember, we all stumble, every one of us.
That's why it's a comfort to go hand in hand.
—EMILY KIMBROUGH

About seven years ago, I had a mother bring her fourth grade son into our office. He had been diagnosed as severely developmentally delayed and was on an array of medications, including lithium. I remember the appointment distinctly because the boy was so out of control that he defecated on the floor of the appointment room. I recommended a number of different things she might try, and she went away with a new arsenal of healthy tools to help her son.

About a year or so ago the mom and I crossed paths, and I asked her about her son. She looked at me, and tears welled up in her eyes. "Dr. Pete," she said, her words filled with emotion, "after two months of coming to you, he was off lithium. A few months later he was off all of his medications. He's now in tenth grade, and he's been off any kind of medication this entire time. He's no longer in special-needs classes; in fact, he's in honors classes and getting As and Bs. He also just completed his Eagle Scout requirements."

Now, there is no guarantee that everyone will transform this remarkably by following our simple lifestyle changes; and clearly we aren't experts in learning disabilities. I do however want you to know that the change in this young man was not the most remarkable thing we've seen in the last 13 years. When our bodies get what they need, remarkable things happen.

The truth is, this boy didn't have a learning disability; his body was overwhelmed by toxic stressors, and it was merely adapting physiologically to the stress that had been placed on his systems for years. One of the greatest stressors was the food he'd been eating. If, instead of putting more stress on our systems by denying them the nutrition they need, we were to empower our bodies to adapt and recover as they were designed to do, we would see miraculous results—just like those seen in this young man.

If this mother had never sought a second opinion for her son in our office, he may have gone through his entire school life dramatically underachieving and causing his family grief and endless anxiety. Instead, when she connected with the right information from a transformational paradigm instead of a classic medical paradigm, things changed for the better—and they changed quickly! Here are some connections you can make to get yourself or your loved ones on a similar road to healthier, happier living.

#1) CONNECT WITH YOUR LOVED ONES

As you prepare for your 21-day Reboot, it is a great idea to connect with your family and those who care the most about you.

First of all, you will need their support and accountability; but more importantly, it may be a great opportunity for you to be an example to them of what getting healthy looks like. Not all families are supportive of each member, but even if your family is not always encouraging to you, this will be a good opportunity to be encouraging to them. You might even save someone's life in the long run!

"Hey Doc, both of my grandparents died from cancer. Is it a given that I will also contract this dreaded disease?"

You may have a genetic predisposition for certain diseases, but that does not mean you are certain to suffer from those diseases. Research now shows us that genetics is only one small piece of the puzzle. We now know that your lifestyle is the most determinant factor in whether you will succumb to disease or not. That means that your environment and your habits have a great deal to do with how your genes express themselves. The choices you make each and every day will determine your health now and in the future, because they determine your environment and how healthfully you choose to live.

At the same time, please don't badger them about what you have read in this book or what you have been taught at one of our meetings. I'm sure they hear all kinds of new theories about diet and healthcare every day. Instead, just talk with them about what you are planning, and ask for their support. Talk to them about the dietary restrictions you will have when you visit them, and what they can expect if they come over to your house for a meal. Don't make a big deal out of it, though, or be offended if they act like it is a hardship to meet your new dietary restrictions. Remember that you want to be an example to them, and the results you achieve will speak for themselves. Your greatest statement will be the walk you walk, not the talk you talk.

#2) CONNECT WITH ALLIES

This is not a battle to fight all alone. Keep in mind what we shared in the last chapter about how those who worked with others at Saddleback Church lost twice the weight of those who followed the program alone. Put the power of teamwork and mutual support on your side!

At the very least, find a friend with whom you can connect and who won't mind your calling for support every day over your first few weeks of the program. If you can, find two friends—one who has been eating healthy for a while, and one who is starting about the same time as you are.

Begin to plug in to our online community or one of the Unhealthy Anonymous chapters around the country. Studies show that people who are in relationship with other people experiencing the same things in life have significantly decreased levels of stress. We are designed to relate to others and walk out life together. Every time you come you will learn new, valuable information firsthand. There is no better way to keep you on track and focused on making your vision a reality.

The ideas we give you in the 12-step program are like seeds that will bring the harvest of a healthy and happy life. But those seeds don't have a chance unless they are grown in the rich, fertile soil of a supportive, nonjudgmental community. This type of community that takes you as you are and helps you get what you want out of life sustains and supports the new growth we are working toward, and I can't stress enough how important it is for you to get plugged in by coming to weekly meetings, attending special events, or even by taking advantage of our online opportunities to connect.

#3) CONNECT WITH A BETTER PARADIGM

Modern medicine today is disease-oriented, not health-oriented. That's not because doctors are evil—many of my friends are doctors, and they are some of the most compassionate and caring people I know. For crisis situations and emergency care, clinics and hospitals are still the best places in the world to be. But the medical profession has the wrong "glasses" on when it comes to keeping people healthy. The diseases that plague us today are quite different from the diseases that were killing people at the dawn of the 20th century. The problem is medical professionals today are still being trained in the thinking of that era—in the time when infectious disease was the greatest threat to human life, something very different from the chronic lifestyle diseases that kill roughly 80 percent of people today.

WAKE-UP CALL

The greatest threat to humans today is that of chronic lifestyle illness. The bubonic plague of the 14th century killed at least 30 percent of the European population, but today 80 percent of the humans in the industrial world suffer with some sort of chronic—or lifestyle—illness.

You see, the greatest medical breakthrough to date came with the advent of antibiotics in the midst of World War II.[1] Why was this so important? Because at that time the greatest killers were diseases that infected the body—generally through individual microbes. Dr. Mark Hyman describes the period:

> Imagine a time before antibiotics when women died of simple childbirth fever, when a bad chest infection could lead to death, when a strep throat caused heart failure, when limbs were amputated because of an infected wound. Those commonplace occurrences seem unimaginable now.[2]

Before the advent of antibiotics, a mere fever could be a sign of the presence of a life-threatening illness, and doctors knew very little about how to save their patients beyond hoping and waiting. Then there was the breakthrough discovery that infectious diseases usually had a common cause—a microbe—and they could be treated with a common remedy—some form of antibiotic. This led medical science to the conclusion that there had to be a pill for every ill—and for a long time that seemed to be right. As Dr. Jeffrey Bland put it in his book, *The Disease Delusion*, "Precisely because it derives from germ theory, it is based in reductionist thinking: find the bug and nuke it with a drug developed for just that purpose. Period."[3] Over the next four generations, pharmaceutical antibiotics and other medications contributed to a near doubling of life expectancy.

The chronic diseases of today, however, are very different from the infectious diseases of yesteryear. Some also call these "lifestyle" diseases, because they seem to have more to do with our environment and habits than with our genetic predispositions. Chronic or lifestyle diseases include type 2 diabetes, cardiovascular diseases, cancer, digestive disorders, dementia, allergies, arthritis, asthma, Parkinson's, autism, hormonal issues, fibromyalgia, chronic fatigue syndrome, attention deficit disorders, depression, and autoimmune deficiencies, along with other ailments that could fit into these categories. None of these diseases is created by a single cause—like a unique type of microbe. Infectious diseases were named after the things that caused them— measles, cholera, pneumonia, smallpox, etc. Chronic diseases are called that because they are chronic— long-lasting, always present, habitual. They are called *chronic* because they attach themselves to us, and then stay until they eventually kill us. These chronic diseases are really more descriptions of a constellation of symptoms than a name that defines the cause of the illness—and no two of these "constellations" are quite the same.

WAKE-UP CALL

Dementia is defined as any severe decline in mental ability. It affects one out of every three senior citizens in North America. The most common type of dementia is Alzheimer's disease.

Currently more than five million Americans are living with Alzheimer's. It is the sixth leading cause of death in our country today. Studies show that overconsumption of grains and sugars increase the risk of Alzheimer's disease. In fact, it is called "Type 3 Diabetes" in some circles.

My father's heart disease is different from your father's. Your aunt's Crohn's disease is different from the Crohn's disease of your neighbor's uncle. What makes them different is that the causes behind each of the symptoms are different. The constellations of contributing factors that lead to each disease are unique for each person. Therefore, because we can't identify a single causal microbe for each, neither can we prescribe a specific medication or combination of medications.

Rather than recognizing these constellations and confronting the issues causing the symptoms, modern medicine focuses on the symptoms themselves and prescribes medications to reduce or eliminate those symptoms. Can you see how that is missing the point? We would be better off digging down one or two layers deeper and trying to discover the cause of the symptoms. Is high blood pressure, for example, being caused by inflammation in the body? If so, is the inflammation being caused by a leaky gut? Or is it coming from a micronutrient deficiency? Maybe a gluten intolerance? Or is increased stress in the person's life from a new job with a hostile work environment the real culprit? Is it perhaps a combination of these factors? Until you can address the true underlying causes, anything else is merely masking the symptoms. If I stumbled across a garbage dump full of waste and junk, there is a good chance that this would eventually become infested with all kinds of bugs and rats. Modern medicine wants to kill the rats and bugs and spray deodorizer so nothing stinks anymore. The problem is the bugs, rats, and rotting smell will return unless that dump gets cleaned up.

This realization is at the dawn of the next great breakthrough in health awareness—"functional medicine." Functional medicine is beginning to change the way we look at the world of illness and wellness. It is a topic we will delve into more deeply in the chapters to come.

YOU HAVE AN ADVOCATE

As you read this book, I want you to know you have people in your corner. My objective in writing this book and helping to create Unhealthy Anonymous is to be an advocate for you, to help you get healthy and stay healthy, to lead you on a journey that will make you stronger and more focused, and to walk with you side by side as you seek to live a life of influence and joy.

Once again, we're not saying we have all of the answers. This is a quest for answers we are on together. We did not start Unhealthy Anonymous to judge others, to condemn them, or to act like know-it-alls. We are on your side. Simply know that I've made many, many mistakes myself, and I am hoping to save others from making those same mistakes when it comes to health, fitness, and overall well-being.

The information in this book is what I have shared with over 1,000,000 people from around the world over the last 13 years; and it has helped them, even though Knoxville, Tennessee is the least likely place for people to come and get good health advice, as it is consistently ranked among the unhealthiest cities in the United States! I know these principles work, because we have heard testimony after testimony from our patients whose lives have been dramatically transformed. These are principles that you too can use to get healthy and stay healthy.

Come as you are, and join with us in this movement to change the conversation about health in America—and more specifically about the enemy of stress that is killing us! I don't care if you have Twizzlers in your pocket and Skittles in your mouth. I know that if you join with friends in Unhealthy Anonymous, read the materials, connect with an ever-growing online community, and come to the meetings, the information we share will help you. You will find a better way to eat and live, and it will make a difference in your family for generations to come.

NOTES

1. Many even say that it made the difference for the Allies in the war, because it saved so many soldiers' lives.

2. Hyman and Jeffrey S. Bland, *The Disease Delusion*, (New York: Harper Wave, 2014), ix.

3. Ibid.,

Step Three

Choose

> But until a person can say deeply and
> honestly, "I am what I am today because
> of the choices I made yesterday," that
> person cannot say, "I choose otherwise."
> —STEPHEN R. COVEY

When I learned that Brian Starkey, one of the contestants from Season 3 of *The Biggest Loser*, was the husband of one of my patients, I asked her if it would be okay if I got his story for this book. I wanted to learn about his experience on the show, as well as his ability to leave the show but still go on to lose more than any of the other contestants who had been eliminated that season. During that time period, he lost more than half his body weight, going from 308 pounds to 152. That is quite an accomplishment! I saw this as an excellent opportunity to learn what works and what doesn't when it comes to long-term weight loss.

Brian's a competitive guy. He grew up as an athlete, and knows what it is like to train and be in shape. He admitted that when he was on the show and he got down to 190 pounds, he should have stopped losing weight at that point. That was a healthy place for him to be, but because he had to lose the most weight to win, he kept going. His weight-loss plan was based on reducing the number of calories he took in through eating, and maximizing the number of calories burned through exercise. To get down to 152 pounds, he worked out for an hour and a half in the morning, an hour at lunch, and then another two hours in the evening. He stayed away from lifting weights, because muscle is heavier than fat, and did a lot of cardio. As you can well imagine, it is not a method he suggests for getting to a healthy weight. Instead, he advocates something more long term and nutritionally focused:

> Being on the show was goal-oriented. It was under the veil of health, but it was really goal oriented, weight-loss oriented, and I pushed to the extreme because I wanted to win....
>
> I sacrificed a lot to get down to that weight, and I don't think it was healthy or good for my relationship with my wife and twin daughters—at least it wouldn't have been if I had kept that up long term.... Thank goodness the show was only a couple of months....
>
> Now I would never be critical of *The Biggest Loser*— I'm incredibly grateful for having the chance to do it. I learned a lot, and they took very good care of us. But you have to recognize that while it is reality TV, it's not reality. It's entertainment; it's there to show people what they can do if they put their minds to it, and it's hyper-accelerated. Health looks totally different what

you see through the window of what *The Biggest Loser* can show you, because the whole thing lasts only eight months.... That show was a time frame, but health is a lifetime.

I also asked Brian how his picture of health and weight loss had changed over the years since the show. If he were going to do it again, what would he do differently? In fact, now that he knows that he purposefully dropped below what was a healthy weight for himself, what would he do now if he wanted to drop 30 pounds or so? He told me *he wouldn't focus on weight loss, but on being healthy*. He described it this way:

If I am eating mostly organic produce—more vegetable based than fruit—grass-fed meats, wild-caught fish, cutting out most of the dairy, and getting the vitamins and micronutrients I need instead of eating processed and fast foods...I will be healthier. If I'm healthier, then maintaining the right weight isn't such an issue, because I will be healthy on a cellular level.... It's not whether or not the food will help me lose weight, the question is, "Is this food going to replenish my body? Will it replenish my cells, or will it kill them?" I like that approach. It makes my choices easier.... For me, total health is first and foremost about food choices....

If, after doing that for a while, I still don't weigh what I want, then it is just a matter of portion control, how often I eat, and maybe adding a little extra exercise for a time. It's not a huge change. It has to be something I can maintain. It should really be about long-term health, not just about weight loss.... The important question shouldn't be "How much weight did I lose since yesterday?" but "Am I getting better—getting healthier—every day?" If I'm not getting my body prepared for the future, for aging, for playing with my kids, for playing with my grandkids even, then I think there is something wrong with my mindset. I might succeed, but it won't be at the things that are really important....

The goal would be to find that sweet spot of maintaining health and creating a baseline for what is a safe range of weight to maintain.... It really comes down to having a plan for living healthy and making choices according to that plan.

THE POWER OF CHOICE

Your ability to choose is a force that can change the world, but it doesn't always feel that way. Many of us feel trapped in the habits and patterns we have practiced over the years. They have become our "normal," and they control what we do at what time throughout the day, how we interact with others, how we organize our lives, and when and how we eat. Willpower is great, but it only goes so far. As John Ortberg once wrote, "Habits eat willpower for breakfast."

I know this is true, because I have seen it and experienced it myself. I remember a new UA member who was sicker than any 28-year-old should ever be. She wanted to change, was motivated to change, and believed in everything we had to offer her. Her plan after talking with a homeopathic doctor and a nutritionist was to cut out all dairy, wheat, and sugar.

She was on the phone telling her grandmother the awesome news that her lung cancer, fibromyalgia, anxiety attacks, panic disorder, arthritis, and obesity could all be solved naturally without any more toxic drugs and radiation. While she was talking on the phone, I watched her unconsciously go into the refrigerator, pull out leftover pizza, heat it in the microwave, and pour herself a tall, cold coke before she even knew what she was doing. When she got off the phone she looked down at the "food," and said, "Well, I guess I'll start this program tomorrow!"

The power of habits—for good or bad—is that we do them unconsciously. Habits take routine activities and turn them into automatic processes so we can spend our intellectual time contemplating other things while we do them. Take, for example, tying your shoes. Do you remember how hard that was at first? When you first started tying your shoes for yourself, you fumbled and restarted constantly until you got it right. Now, when is the last time you thought, "Okay, I have to cross these two ends and pull that tight, make a rabbit ear, and then…"? Probably not since a week after the first time you ever tied your shoes, right?

When we are learning any new task, we can be categorized in one of four learning groups:

1. **The unconsciously incompetent.** These are the people who don't know; but they don't even know that they don't know! A lot of people are blinded by our "super-sized" cultural standards of what nutrition is, and they don't even know what real health looks like. (You may have been like that before you picked up this book, but hopefully that is changing quickly!)

2. **The consciously incompetent.** These are the people who realize there is a need for change, even though

they may not know what that change needs to be. They realize there are skills and habits they don't have, and they want to develop them; but they also know they are far from being very good at these new skills and habits.

3. **The consciously competent.** These are the people who are starting to form the right habits, but have to remind themselves every day to stay with the program. They have to consciously think of the techniques they are trying to master, and they still need to write down every step of the daily routine they are trying to create.

4. **The unconsciously competent.** These are the people whose habits have become so natural that they don't have to think about them consciously to do them. This is "spontaneous right action," and this is the level we want everyone to get to with regard to the 12 steps of this program.

Now think about this in relationship to the first time you drove to work or the grocery store in your new neighborhood. Maybe you had a map or put the address into the GPS on your phone the first time, but now it is so automatic and second nature that you can actually sort through most of the events of your day on the way there, make a phone call, sing along with the radio, and still arrive without a thought to your destination. This is the same process that happens when you stop at the coffee shop to get a latte with whipped cream and a Danish every morning, or that spurs you to get up from your desk as soon as the clock hits 10 AM to go to the break room and buy a diet soda and a candy bar for some quick energy. It's also the thing that makes having seconds feel normal, or doing exercise feel abnormal. We are creatures of habit, and many of those habits are counterproductive.

"Hey Doc, diet soda has to be better for me than regular soda, right?"

No, it is actually worse! Artificial sweeteners are dangerous, addictive excitotoxins that cause excessive firing of neurons and encourage cell death. They also trigger the insulin response just as sugar does and still cause weight gain. But because they have no calories, they leave your hormones more confused than ever!

Bad habits make changing our lives difficult, because they are ingrained patterns that resist change as violently as our immune system resists disease. Our unconscious minds feel safe and comfortable in our habits, and we are wired for self-preservation, which loves safety and comfort. It can seem like a gargantuan effort to change a habit—so much so that many of us give up after just a couple of tries.

However, if you know about how habits really work, how they are created, and how they are broken, then you can turn the tables on bad habits, recreate them from the inside out by making conscious choices, and before you know it—usually in just three weeks or so—your habits will have changed to the point that you are no longer a slave to them, but have instead put them to work for you.

CHANGE YOUR ROUTINES

In his book, *The Power of Habit*, Charles Duhigg explains that habits are made of three parts. First there is a *cue*, some event that has happened regularly enough over time that you have a normal reaction to it, like putting on your shoes before going outside or drive to work. That is followed by the *routine*—the thing you do without thinking in response to the cue, like actually tying your shoes. Then there is the *reward*—your shoes are tied and your feet stay warm and dry. Our life has thousands of these little habit cycles that we have formed over the years—most of them created unconsciously.

WAKE-UP CAL

Aspartame is an artificial sweetener used in over 6,000 products worldwide. This includes many "healthy" products like some low-fat, low-calorie yogurts.

The good news is that because all habits are learned, then they can also be unlearned. It may be more accurate to say that a better habit can be learned in its place. Once we are aware that we have a bad habit and we recognize the *cue* that sets the habit into motion, we suddenly have new power. This allows us to engage our conscious brains to choose a different *routine* in response to the *cue* and receive a more desirable *reward*. Once we do that enough times—the usual time frame for this is recognized as 21 days for things we do daily—we replace the old habit with a more desirable one. Over time, this practice allows us to retool our lives and create habits that will take us automatically in any direction we want to go. To make such a choice means to make a decision. *Decision* literally means "to cut." When you decide something, you are choosing one option and deciding to *cut away* all others. It means you are focusing your energies and attention in your chosen direction and ignoring every other direction.

The same thing happens when you set a goal within your vision for better health. Say you have decided that you would like to be able to run again. You watch people lining up for the Turkey Trot, or some other 5K event, and a little voice in the back of your mind says, "I wish I could do that someday." Usually you shush that voice, but today you realize that it is the most unique and authentic part of you. You don't shush it with rational reasons why you will never run again; instead you listen to it, you honor it, and you decide to make some changes in your life. You cast the vision of what it will be like when you can actually run 10 steps, then a quarter mile, then a 5K. You check with your doctor and use common sense to set up a training program. And you ease into it one little step at a time. You set your goal: Next year at this time I will be able to run a quarter of a mile without collapsing. And you begin. After all, next year will come and go—you may as well be closer to your goal!

UNDERSTANDING EMOTIONAL ATTACHMENTS TO FOOD

Sometimes the habits we form around food aren't haphazard or random. There can be very deep emotional and psychological issues connected to why we eat as we do. Some are even the results of traumas we experienced when we were younger. Such issues can be deep-seated and painful to confront. This is why, in addition to connecting with family members and a support group, it is also a good idea to connect with a counselor or psychologist if you feel like your habits have far more control over you than you think they should.

We all have needs to feel secure, to belong, and to feel loved; and much of what we do to protect those needs will be unconscious and integrally entwined with our relationship to food. Sometimes traumas from our childhood can make being overweight a psychological protective shield or barrier to keep trauma away. We feel as if being "unattractive" will keep predators away from us. Others will go to the opposite extreme, refusing to eat because they believe they are fat when no one else thinks so, or getting stuck in cycles of binging and starving themselves and then hating themselves for their lack of self-control.

Some who eat when they are stressed or depressed feel as if they have no control over events in their lives. In this case, food can be a fast track to feeling better. There is a reason, after all, some foods are called "comfort food." Those who do this feel better until the guilt sets in about the amount or type of food they have just consumed. The next response is often despair—"I've already blown it, so I may as well eat the whole thing."

There are dozens of different scenarios for how this takes place, and the best way to deal with these issues is to talk them through with a professional counselor, create strategies to deal with the root causes of these patterns, and to find better ways of dealing with the emotional and psychological cues that are sabotaging your efforts to create the life you really want. Confronting the underlying issues and regaining control of your life is not an easy process, but it's definitely worth it. The important thing is to make choices about your life that are in line with your vision of what you want your life to look like. Then get rid of anything that doesn't align with that vision. You are not stuck in a rut! You have the power of choice each moment of each and every day!

Regaining control doesn't mean you won't fall back into old habit patterns from time to time. Sometimes you will be too hungry, you won't plan well for the day, or you will merely decide you are going to choose to follow an old habit rather than the new one you want to form. That happens. We all fall down from time to time, but the key is to get back up again.

CHOOSE TO STACK THE DECK IN YOUR FAVOR

As you probably know, one of the biggest issues with changing your eating is that people get too hungry to stay on a restrictive plan, and their cravings for certain foods make them cheat. Then, when they don't get the results they want, they give up out of frustration.

The way to avoid these pitfalls is to change your appetite and satisfy your hunger with highly-nutritional, good-fat foods that will switch off your hunger signals and make handling cravings much more manageable. When you begin to heal your gut biome, you will find that cravings disappear. In addition, you need to have a plan for how to replace your normal routines when it comes to craving cues. Replace candy with fruit, for example, or a handful of almonds. If you are tired and hungry, go exercise instead of grazing through your kitchen for snacks. If you have a number of better responses for cues that usually tempt you to eat the wrong things, it's just a matter of choosing a new routine in response to the old cue. As you do, you will form new habits and respond to your cravings with better foods or activities.

The foods that are the best for us are more a symphony than a solo act. While our body breaks down what we eat into components to digest it, macronutrients (proteins, fats, and carbohydrates) and micronutrients (vitamins, trace minerals, and organic acids) need each other in combination to be absorbed effectively by our bodies. By divine design, whole, real foods have complimentary combinations of macro- and micronutrients built in to ensure we get the maximum absorption of the nutrients from each bite we eat. Processed foods, on the other hand, may try to combine macro- and micronutrients to make them sound healthy, but your body knows it isn't getting the real deal. Enriched (adding nutrients back in that were removed in processing) or fortified (adding vitamins or minerals that were never there before) foods are poor counterfeits of the combinations that occur in real foods.

DID YOU KNOW?

Omega-3 deficiency is a common, often overlooked, underlying cause of cancer.

It's sort of like the difference between lightning and a lightning bug. We may say, "Oh, look at that beautiful display by the lightning bugs!" But we know that they really don't contain lightning. Lightning bugs are attractive, but lightning is powerful!

Your body is in the habit of adapting to the conditions around it, and it is always trying to determine if you are living through a feast or a famine. The thing is, this isn't determined by the quantity of food you eat; it's determined by the quality. Your body is looking for what it can digest and use, and it could care less about what is just passing on through. So, if you eat a moderate or small quantity of nutrient-dense foods, what happens? Your body isn't hungry between meals. Eat massive amounts of nutrient-empty foods and what happens? Your body calls out, "Mayday, mayday! We're starving to death in here! Eat more!"

Most processed foods are essentially *carb*-board with all of the value leached out through processing. They are made to taste good and be addictive through added flavor enhancers and the right mixture of salt, bad fats, sugar, and bad carbohydrates (sugar in disguise). These drug and take advantage of your taste buds while giving few if any life-sustaining combinations of macro- and micronutrients to your body. The end effect is they are empty calories that leave you craving more.

WAKE-UP CALL

The estimated annual medical cost of obesity in the U.S. was $147 billion in 2008 U.S. dollars; the medical costs for people who are obese were $1,429 higher than those of normal weight.

Your body then either stores the "solo-act" nutrients in the hope of trying to digest them later when it gets the right complimentary nutrients, or it adds them into the ever-lengthening queue of items to be flushed. At the same time, it sends out the alert. "Hey! We need more nutrients down here!" So what do you grab? More than likely, the same tasty, nutrient-poor foods you love because they've been chemically enhanced and manipulated to hit the "bliss point" of your taste buds. That's the reason "You can't eat just one!" These are foods that have been molecularly-engineered to hit your taste buds just right, to turn on your hunger mechanisms and encourage you to graze and snack all day long. All the while your systems are stressed, and they begin to adapt physiologically by sending out warning signals in the form of symptoms. At this point, many will go to a doctor and get medication to suppress those unwelcome or uncomfortable symptoms instead of treating them as the wonderful messengers they are! Your symptoms are trying to tell you something. Are you listening?

What if you took your car in to the mechanic because the oil light kept flashing—maybe it was flashing at random times—maybe not all the time, but enough of the time to annoy you and distract you from your main purpose of driving to work. Then what if the mechanic told you, "I have just the thing to fix that!" as he took a nice small square of black electrical tape and carefully applied it to that nasty, flashing, and irritating oil light. Would you say, "Ah...that's better!" Or would you get a new mechanic? Yes! You would get a new mechanic and then probably report that old mechanic to the Better Business Bureau! Why do we treat our bodies any differently? They are flashing warnings at us to tell us something. When we go for advice to a highly educated, highly trained professional, what we are given is the careful application of a scientifically researched, peer-reviewed, FDA approved, over-priced square of "electrical tape"!

The best example of this "electrical tape" approach is the current overuse of statin drugs. For the past six decades, medical authorities have warned us that saturated animal fats cause heart disease and should be severely restricted in a heart-healthy diet. But is that really the whole truth? An important editorial written by an interventional cardiology specialist in the British Medical Journal states that the whole "saturated fat consumption causes heart disease" is a myth.[1] Reducing saturated fat intake reduces large, buoyant (type A) LDL particles. But it's the small, dense (type B) particles that are implicated in heart disease, and these respond to reductions in carbohydrate consumption. A high-sugar diet raises your risk for heart disease by promoting metabolic syndrome—a cluster of health conditions, including high blood pressure, insulin resistance (pre-diabetic condition), high triglycerides, and the accumulation of fat around your vital organs.[2] In order to reverse or avoid insulin resistance, you need to avoid (as much as possible) sugar, fructose, grains, and processed foods; eat whole foods; and replace the grain carbs with high quality healthful fats like coconut oil, avocados, raw dairy, organic whole eggs, and organic grass-fed butter.

BETTER CHOICES WILL LEAD TO A BETTER YOU!

The frontal lobe of the human brain is the center of personality and emotion. It is also in charge of decision making. Most of the dopamine-sensitive neurons found in the neural sheath that covers the brain are found in the frontal lobe. The dopamine system is in charge of reward, attention, short-term memory, performing tasks, planning, and motivation. The frontal lobe also directs impulse control, aggression, hunger, sexual drive, spatial relations, and language comprehension. All of these variants play into our ability to make wise choices; indeed into our basic intention and motivation to make and stick to the choices we have made when things get difficult—especially when faced with the choice of denying immediate pleasure for the sake of future reward. This is an ability that animals don't have. It is what makes us able to do the incredible things that human beings do.

What gives the frontal cortex such power is its ability to recognize patterns in our behavior, determine that there are actions we can take to deny short-term pleasure for the sake of long-term satisfaction, and then step into that pattern and choose differently that we might eventually become unconsciously competent at doing the right things. This is how we change our habits, and then those changed habits change our quality of life.

Some choices and strategies that might "make or break" your success in this program are not that different from choices and strategies that you would adopt if you went to drug or alcohol rehab.

1.   **Make a chart** with the benefits of living as you are now on one side, and the benefits of changing what you are doing on the other side. Keep this as a visual reminder of why you are changing. For example, if eating pasta and pizza is really fun for you, and hard to let go of, make a chart for that one behavior. On the left would be, "It tastes good." On the right would be five or ten reasons to stop.

2.   **Make a list** of people and places that aren't safe for you. Then avoid those people and those places. If you are trying to avoid drinking alcohol, you don't plan to have dinner at a sports bar. It's just too dangerous, and it almost guarantees failure. Likewise, if you are trying to change your ability to control portions, you don't go to an "all you can eat" restaurant. That is a recipe for disaster. If Aunt Matilda is a food pusher, or there is nothing "safe" to eat at your friend Jim's house, then guess what? You should avoid those people while you are trying to build new habits.

3.   **Learn from past mistakes.** Every saint has a past, and every sinner has a future. We've all made mistakes, and lived to regret them. When someone tries to remind you of who you used to be, or reminds you of all the times you've tried to change before, just look at them humbly and say, "By God's grace, it will be different this time." When it's the man or woman in the mirror who is beating you down because you went totally off the reservation, look at that person and humbly ask, "What can I learn from this experience that will make me stronger next time??" And don't be afraid to start again tomorrow. That's why they say, "One day at a time."

4. Remember to H.A.L.T. That stands for "hungry, angry, lonely, or tired." When we are in a state of deprivation from being hungry, angry, lonely, or tired, we easily slip back into unconscious choices and habits that are unproductive at best, destructive at worst. Practice self-care so that you don't get into a state of deprivation that sets you up for failure in your program of health. If you feel yourself in one of those states, remedy it as quickly as possible and move on. Eat a snack, breathe deeply and take a walk, call a friend or mentor, give and get a hug, or take a nap. Take care of yourself.

Once again, I hope you see the importance of these first three steps of Unhealthy Anonymous—

1. **Identify** the enemy.

2. **Connect** with others and the right paradigm to gain advantage in fighting that enemy.

3. **Choose** the right strategies for conquering and containing the enemy.

These three steps set the stage for long-term success using the power of choosing wisely as the fulcrum. The right knowledge and understanding helps you make an informed strategy, but it also equips, empowers, and motivates you as you walk out that strategy in your everyday life. When you understand that stress is the real enemy, then you can know you aren't just shadow boxing. This knowledge leads to an informed strategy with which to plan your attack, and when you act on the plan and start to see incremental improvement, your resolve snowballs toward living a life aligned with the purpose and the vision of how you want to live—you enter the gates of "happy and healthy," and you laugh at anyone suggesting you should go back to the way things were before.

EVOLUTION VS. REVOLUTION

Step 1: Cereal with milk each morning
Step 2: Cereal with almond milk each morning
Step 3: Healthy fats and proteins for breakfast

Remember as well: this is a marathon, not a sprint. You are better off starting slowly and finding a maintainable pace than jumping in with some radical program and burning out like a sugar crash. My hope is that the principles you find here will keep you healthy and energized for a long time—well into your 80s, 90s, and beyond!

Now that we have dealt with the intellectual and emotional decision steps, it's time to move on to the other steps of this program that will enable you to start making the desired changes in your life. That all starts with recognizing the most underrated health problem of our modern, industrial, information age—the problem of chronic stress.

NOTES

1. Aseem Malhotra, "Saturated Fat Is Not the Major Issue," TheBMJ, May 15, 2014, doi:http://dx.doi.org/10.1136/bmj.f6340.

2. Dr. Mercola, "Saturated Fat Does Not Promote Heart Disease," Mercola.com, November 4, 2013, http://articles.mercola.com/sites/articles/archive/2013/11/04/saturated-fat-intake.aspx.

Recognize

Until the enemy is exposed, we
will never get the victory!
—DR. PETE

The human body has been designed to
resist an infinite number of changes and
attacks brought about by its environment.
The secret of good health lies in successful
adjustment to changing stresses on the body.
—DR. HARRY J. JOHNSON

Annette looked forward to her new contract as a project man-
ager with mixed feelings. It was a great opportunity for her
to advance her career, but she also knew the level of stress that
accompanies this kind of a position, and what that would mean
for her health.

You see, Annette had been diagnosed with Crohn's disease in 1995 when she was 35. Though she had managed it fairly well over the last 17 years, the flare-ups would all but knock her out—flu-like symptoms, pain in her lower gastrointestinal tract, and little to no energy. At the same time, managing it meant taking nine pills a day at a cost of $600 a month. Each new drug she was prescribed—from Asacol to Flagyl to Predisone to Remicade—came with its own set of life-complicating side effects. Not only that, but when she was stressed, no matter what medications she was on, she would still experience flare-ups.

As it turned out, the stress from the new job had horrible results on her Crohn's—even worse than she had anticipated. Annette became desperate for a better answer. While driving down the road with her husband, she saw our sign and decided to drop in. Her husband's back had been hurting, and they decided to give us a try. During their visit, I was able to share with Annette's husband our philosophy about keeping people healthy as opposed to treating chronic symptoms with pills, shots, surgery, or antidepressants. He signed his wife up for an appointment before he left the building.

When Annette came in to see me, she told me about her Crohn's disease, and I told her that my good friend Jordan Rubin had experienced many of the same effects of this chronic disease as well. Jordan had even been near death as a result, but had cured it by changing his diet. I told her about his new book, *The Maker's Diet Revolution*. She was floored. She had been given a copy of Jordan's original book, *The Maker's Diet*, by a friend shortly after it had come out, read most of it, ordered some of his supplements that he recommended for Crohn's disease, but had never actually tried the diet. She felt like it was by the grace of God we'd met, and she was reminded of Jordan's diet solution.

WAKE-UP CALL

A new survey shows that more than eight in ten employed Americans are stressed out by at least one thing about their jobs. Poor pay and increasing workloads were top sources of concern reported by American workers. Fourteen percent of workers reported low paychecks as their main source of work-related stress. And this is in America—one of the richest countries in the world!

Fourteen percent also ranked a heavy workload as the top stressor—up nine percent from 2013. These concerns were followed by frustration with coworkers or commutes (both eleven percent), working in a job that is not one's career of choice (eight percent), poor work-life balance (seven percent), lack of opportunity for advancement (six percent), and fear of being fired or laid off (four percent).

A few months later, we brought Jordan in to speak at one of our meetings, and both Annette and her husband attended. At the time we were offering a 14-day "Get Well" plan for anyone who wanted to try the diet. Annette signed up. She also secretly decided that she would stop taking her Crohn's medications when she started the diet just to see what would happen. She knew she might have to start them again if the flare-ups returned, but she wanted to give her body a chance to totally detox while she treated her condition with real foods alone.

The good news is, since that day Annette has never returned to any of her medications—she has never even needed one pill. Not only that, but after the 14-day plan, she felt better than she had ever hoped she would. As she put it in a letter to us about her experience:

I feel so blessed to be on this path to wellness. I pray
a prayer of thanks every day. Not only does my family notice a difference in me; my longtime friends are
amazed at how much I have changed. I will be ever
grateful to Dr. Pete and Jordan Rubin for the rest of
my life.

Annette, like so many people we have worked with, recognized
that it wasn't enough to just identify she had a problem—she also
needed to recognize the true underlying cause of that problem—
stress—and give her body what it needed to be able adapt to and
recover from it.

The greatest problem with the medical paradigm today is that
they are conditioned and trained to address symptoms, not get to
the real root of the problem. Many see disease as multifaceted and
complicated, but the truth is that beneath all symptoms there is
really one main root cause of the lifestyle diseases we are facing
today, and most symptoms grow out of it. If we are going to get to
real health, we have to address the biggest problem, and we have
to recognize that at the root of all chronic disease is the very real,
modern problem of *stress*.

A PARADIGM FOR SICKNESS OR A PARADIGM FOR HEALTH?

Since the beginning of the medical profession, what kind of
people have gone to see doctors? Sick people—people who are having medical problems or an emergency of some kind or another.
The challenge to doctors has always been not to help the healthy
maintain that condition, but to make the sick better. The assump-
tion has always been, "If you feel good; you're healthy. If it's not

broken; don't fix it." So the paradigm for most doctors has always started with disease and the science of how and why people get sick and die. The natural outcome of that paradigm is that if you can get people back to feeling good, then they will be healthy—that if you can alleviate the symptoms, you are staving off the effects of disease, and that person will live longer. Well, it doesn't exactly work that way—especially when it comes to lifestyle diseases like cardiovascular disease, obesity, cancer, diabetes, dementia, and the rest.

WAKE-UP CALL

The American Cancer Society reports that in 2014 alone, 142,000 *new* cancers were reported in citizens under the age of 45!

That's not even taking into account all the cases of cancer in young folks that have *already* been reported and are being currently treated.

You see, optimal health is not getting right up to the edge of what the body can tolerate and then dialing it back a notch so you don't recognize what is really happening inside of you. How many times have you heard of people who worked out, felt great, thought they were in the prime of their lives, even had a good checkup, and then suddenly, as if out of nowhere, they had a heart attack or they got a cancer diagnosis? Unfortunately it happens all of the time. Why? Because, as a rule, before taking them seriously we wait until our "warning signs" are so advanced that the damage is far too great to recover. We assume that whatever we are doing and eating—living sedentary lives; filling our bodies with toxins from alcohol, tobacco, and processed foods; failing to address heavy metals in our systems; carrying too much extra weight; and dealing with too much stress each and every day—is okay until we reach some crisis point marked by our blood sugar level, cholesterol count, or some other indicator in our bodies that things are abnormal. Then we take a pill or treatment to get those levels back within the acceptable range and go on as if the problem had been handled. Meanwhile, whatever we were doing that caused the abnormality in the first place is still in our lives. We have treated the symptoms but have done nothing about the cause.

DID YOU KNOW?

A high blood glucose level (anything over 110 mg/dL) has been indicated in breast cancer—especially in older women.

Only ten percent of breast cancers are genetic. The other 90 percent come as a result of lifestyle—especially exposure to harmful chemicals that stress women's bodies by disrupting hormonal balances.

Doctors judge patients' health by what they call "pathology reports." For example, they look at a pathology report generated by the results of a given blood test. What is *pathology*? According to the *Merriam-Webster Dictionary* it means, "1: the study of the essential nature of diseases and especially of the structural and functional changes produced by them, 2: *something abnormal*." So, by contrast they are defining *healthy* as "the absence of abnormality."

Health is not the absence of abnormality! It is the presence of proper function. But what do the doctors tell you? In essence, they say, "Sure, your immune system may be stressing out, your arteries might be hardening, your cells may not be getting the materials and communication with the brain they need to reproduce properly, and you may be 40 pounds overweight, but your blood work looks good. Maybe you could just eat fewer calories and exercise a little more to get that weight off? Other than that, no need for intervention at this point. See you next year around the same time."

"Hey Doc, why do I need to exercise? I'm too tired; and it hurts!"

Exercise actually eases chronic pain, lowers blood pressure, revs up your metabolism, and helps with insomnia as well as depression.
You need to move to get rid of pain and fatigue!

This is why I've never really liked the pathology paradigm. It is not based on causes, it is based on symptoms, and it assumes that if you cure the symptoms, you have returned the body to normal function and you are out of danger. It's a little like assuming you are okay financially, because not all of your credit cards are maxed out yet. You still have a couple hundred dollars left on one credit card for groceries, so everything is fine. What happens, though, if you lose your job and suddenly have no income? It doesn't take much to push you over the edge and on your way toward bankruptcy.

Let me give you a simple example of why the pathology paradigm is so often giving us the wrong interpretation of the facts. Imagine taking a field trip from our office in Knoxville, Tennessee to Denver, Colorado. It is well known that Denver is the mile-high city, and that the air is thinner at higher altitudes. So, one of the first things that would happen once we stepped off of the airplane is that we would probably be a little short of breath, especially if we exerted ourselves, because thinner air means we have to breathe more to get the same amount of oxygen we did when we were at sea level. So what do our bodies do? They start to create more red blood cells in order to produce more oxygen.

If you just happened to have a doctor right there to do a blood test, you would find out that you have an "abnormal" red blood cell count. Would you consider that increase in red blood cells to be a pathology or an adaption? Your physiology is adapting, of course! Even though your red blood cell count is "abnormal," there isn't anything wrong! Your body is merely adapting physiologically to handle the conditions of your new environment. The increase in red blood cells is, in fact, normal and necessary. It is a sign that your body is doing what it does best—adapting to stimuli so that it can keep itself healthy and operate at peak performance.

Instead of looking at the body as either normal or abnormal—like a light switch that is either on or off—I like to look at the body as an organism always working to heal itself and come to a state of balance and rest. How well is the body succeeding in this important endeavor? *This* is the key to whether or not you are healthy or sick. I call this the *adaptive physiology model* as many innovators in medicine are starting to do. Instead of looking at the body as normal or abnormal, let's look at how the body is adapting to the challenges it is facing, and if it's not adapting well, then why not? When we determine that, we will know better how to help the body heal itself.

The question shouldn't be, "What's abnormal?" but "What do we need to add to the body to help it keep itself healthy, and what do we need to take away from it to keep it from being overtaxed?"

Rather than waiting for a disease to show itself and then addressing the symptoms of that disease, we should focus on keeping the body healthy by giving it everything it needs and protecting it from what hurts it.

WHAT STRESS REALLY DOES TO US

Let me give you another illustration. Let's say we go to the zoo together. It's a beautiful day, and we decide to get out in the sunshine. As we come around the corner to where the big cats are housed, we see people moving quickly in the other direction. We think it is a little odd, but we are talking, so we continue on. As we get to the center of that area, we are struck by the fact that no one is around. Then off to the side we notice a couple of zookeepers creeping forward with a pole that has a rope noose at the end for catching wild animals. "That's weird." Then the workers see us, and their eyes get really big. They are mouthing something to us. What is it? It seems to be just one word, the same word, over and over. It looks like the word… "Run!"

At that moment, we hear a roar and our attention is drawn in the other direction. There, standing just outside of his cage with the door wide open, licking his lips, is the zoo's prized attraction—a Bengal tiger. Just as we see him, we realize he has been watching us the entire time, and has only one thought in his mind: "Lunch."

As the tiger twitches, we spin and run. We don't look back to see if the tiger is following us or not, because we are focused on one thing—getting out of there as quickly as possible!

As we turn and run, our bodies go into what is called fight or flight mode (in this case, we are exercising the flight part). The sympathetic nervous system begins to dictate changes that are beyond our control. Our entire body chemistry changes in a few short seconds. A message goes straight to our adrenal glands to start producing adrenaline, noradrenaline, epinephrine, and nor-ephinephrine. These powerful chemicals increase heart rate and stroke volume to provide more blood to our brains so we can think more clearly, and to our muscles so we can act more quickly and run faster. We suddenly feel more alert and alive as a shot of adrenaline courses through our bodies.

WAKE-UP CALL

In 1908, Dr. Eli Jones published a book entitled *Cancer: Its Causes, Symptoms, and Treatment*. In it, Dr. Jones reveals the top causes of cancer. Do you know what was at the top of his list? *Stress!* [1]

If we knew that over a century ago, why do we pay so little attention to stress today?

Our arteries constrict, raising blood pressure and forcing blood into muscles so we can run, fight, or do whatever is neces-sary. Our spinal cords begin to stretch and lengthen like rubber bands being pulled at both ends— sending even more messages to our brains that there's an emergency at hand. Metabolism is amped up, and the digestive system has shut down. We will feel hungry when this is all over—if we survive, that is—but for now the appetite is a low priority. All the energy our bod-ies would normally use to digest and process food is redirected to only the basic functions necessary for survival. Likewise, the sex drive, immune system, and growth hormone production all shut down to preserve vital energy. This clears communication channels for our bodies to do whatever they need in order to protect themselves from this present danger. Our brains shut down normal learning functions like fact retention and working memory. Logic is inhibited, but emotions and instinct are high. The chemistry of our blood changes by increasing the clotting factors in preparation for any wounds or damages that may occur in the ensuing conflict.[2] Our bodies have gone into crisis mode. We are in an abnormal state.

If at this particularly stressful time a doctor were to take your blood pressure, she would definitely find it elevated! If she were to offer you a pill to bring it back under control, you would look at her as if she were crazy! You don't need a prescription to get back to normal, you need for someone to put that tiger back in its cage! Now you may laugh at this, but that is exactly what is happening in medical offices and hospitals all across the United States every day. People are being chased by the "tiger" of stress, and their doctors are ignoring it and treating what is happening to their bodies as a result of being chased. They are addressing the *pathology*, not the *cause* of the pathology.

Are you beginning to see why this might not always be the best approach?

Recently Glenn Beck, a very famous conservative radio and television host, called his family around him because doctors told him he didn't have much life left in him. He had been experiencing what could only be called a total health crisis when previously he had felt "just fine." Turns out his adrenal glands were shot from stress, and his whole body was following suit. Fortunately, he turned to some alternative methods of health, changing his diet, his lifestyle, and his whole way of relating to the world. Now he is very much alive and back on mission. But the point is that it's not "just stress"! Stress kills! Stress steals! Stress destroys!

THREE STAGES OF STRESS

Our bodies react to stress in three rather distinct phases. One could think of them as levels of alertness in the face of perceived or actual threats. The first stage is a call to "battle stations" in the face of an immediate threat or a need for increased vigilance. It is the state our bodies entered when we realized the tiger wasn't in its cage. It's actually a little like a superpower. Our blood pressure rises; our breathing rate increases, getting more oxygen to our brains and muscles; digestion, immunity, and other systems go on hold to divert energy to systems that will help us either fight or flee; our pupils dilate to see better; hearing increases; all the same things I described in the last section. The short-term effect of this is that we are smarter, faster, and stronger. We are as ready as we can be to engage or get away from whatever the threat may be.

In our modern world, this is seldom staving off an actual attack, though. More likely, it is facing the fear of speaking in front of a group ;dealing with a hostile customer, colleague, or relative; or putting in extra hours and effort to meet a project deadline that is quickly approaching. It could also mean facing a loved one's illness or injury, having difficulty starting a family, facing money pressures, or getting yelled at by your boss. Your body then internally adapts to help you handle that external stimulus. It is a short-term response that puts you in peak performance mode. This is considered phase one of stress, and it is a good thing—but only if it remains a short-term response.

A phase-one stress response can also be set off by a number of internal events. It could be triggered by a virus, by toxins in what you ingest, by a perceived threat that isn't real, or even by expectations you have of yourself that no one else even knows about. It can be brought on by an environment that is polluted, by an injury, by chronically running on little sleep, by being undernourished, by living with guilt or holding a grudge, by burying your emotions instead of dealing with them, by feeling hopeless about the future, drinking too much caffeine, or any number of other things. No matter whether your stress is coming from internal or external factors, if it is prolonged, you will enter phase two of stress.

WAKE-UP CALL

Ten years ago autism affected one in ten thousand children.

The number now is one in 44. New studies show that gut biome is directly linked to this condition.

We were not designed to stay stressed for long periods of time without a break. If stress continues for too long, our bodies enter phase two where they seek to balance their functional needs with the continued need for hyper-alertness. This will mean tradeoffs, imbalances, and fatigued systems. As this continues, you become overtired, irritable, and find it hard to think straight. Sometimes human bodily systems will attack things that they shouldn't. These attacks are responsible for allergies and autoimmune diseases. Sometimes the body will ignore glaring symptoms as if it is just too tired to care. This may cause you to binge eat to deal with the emotions that accompany this stress. Your body will likely store fat as if getting ready for a famine. It may cause you to crash into bed on a Friday night and do little but sleep until you have to get back to work on Monday morning. You can survive this stage for some time—years, in fact—but not without consequences. The longer you stay in phase two of stress, the more repair your systems are going to need when you do finally get a rest. However, if you keep on without that rest, you are going to enter phase three.

"Hey Doc, I can't seem to remember anything anymore. I'm too young to be so forgetful! What can I do?"

Most Americans don't get nearly enough healthy fats, omega-3s, vitamin B_{12} or vitamin D. These substances protect the brain from degeneration and can actually repair previous damage. Chronic stress can cause memory problems, as can toxicity from heavy metals. Eating grains can cause "brain fog."

To protect against this, replace many of your grains with healthy fats and lean protein.

Phase three is exhaustion. You've been running on turbo for way too long. This is where things start to break down from the strain. The body may be filled with inflammation. Mutant cells may metastasize and become cancerous. Blood vessel walls may become rigid and lined with pockets of plaque. These pockets can then burst, causing a heart attack or stroke. The immune system becomes imbalanced and causes any number of health complications. In other words, you have full-blown problems with lifestyle diseases. You might feel just fine—after all, you've been operating like this for years—but on the inside you are on the verge of something serious and life altering.

Now this is the place where a doctor may come in, look at your blood, and say something like, "Your cholesterol is too high. I want to put you on this statin drug," or "Your blood pressure is too high. I have this medication I want you to take *for the rest of your life.*" Do you get a little glimpse of why that might not be address-ing the real issue? It's a little like leaving the tiger out of the cage and saying, "Hey, I'll just put on this blindfold. That way I won't see the tiger anymore. Then my systems should calm down and go back to normal." That wouldn't really solve anything, would it? Isn't it a better idea to just put the tiger back in its cage?

But why don't we think the same thing when we go to a doctor who says, "You have high blood pressure. I'm going to put you on a drug that will lower it." High blood pressure is just an indicator light that something is going on in your body that your body is trying to adapt to. The response shouldn't be, "Well, let's mask this symptom." The response should me, "Hmm, I wonder what could be causing my blood pressure to go up?" When a doctor prescribes a pill, shot, surgery, or antidepressant, they aren't curing anything, they are just putting a little piece of black electrical tape over the indicator light.

Do you now see why people can be put on such medications and still get cancer or have heart attacks? Just as little pieces of black tape will not keep your car's engine from seizing because it has no oil in it, pills, shots, surgery, or antidepressants won't keep your body from falling apart. They won't provide the necessary building blocks for your body to heal itself.

YOU NEED TO PROTECT YOUR ASSETS

A few years ago I was asked by a cancer treatment center to come and speak with some of their leading oncologists. After my address, one of them came up to me and said, "Dr. Pete, you hit the nail on the head."

"What do you mean?" I asked.

"We are spending more money on cancer research in America and in the world than ever before in history," he began, "and yet, cancer rates are skyrocketing exponentially. I think we missed the boat somewhere."

"I would have to agree," I said. "Where did we miss it, in your opinion?"

"Well, I think it's exactly like you said, 'cancer is a stress response,' but since most researchers don't see that, I think we're looking at the wrong studies. Johns Hopkins University recently said that one of every two men and one out of every three women will be diagnosed with cancer in this generation. Today, it feels like everyone knows someone who has cancer, but I don't think the same was true even just ten years ago.

"At the same time, there's another interesting study that tells us we experience more stress in one month today than people did in their entire lifetimes just a generation ago. How can there not be a correlation? If one charts the amount of stress in our society today, he would see that stress levels are increasing at basically the same rate cancer is. Why can't we see that stress *is causing* cancer? We're looking in the wrong places trying to find a pharmaceutical solution to cancer. The big issue is *stress*. We've got to find a way to do something about stress."

Modern society encourages us to live to the very limit of our resources and strength in everything we do. It often demands we spend more than 40 or 50 hours a week at work, that we eat and drink to excess because that is what brings pleasure, and that we zone out in front of the TV or computer every evening to keep up with current events, entertainment, and social network "friends." Many of us spend more time communicating with people we barely know then we do with the people we have actual relation-ships with. We need to realize that these new "norms" are not based on what is best for us and our loved ones, but on a consumer culture that is willing to "spend" our lives for its own benefit. If we are going to choose instead to have happy and healthy lives, we need to recognize that life demands trade-offs and prioritization. We need to recognize stress for the escaped tiger that it is, and learn how to put it back into its cage.

NOTES

1. "Stress Linked to Cancer," Mercola.com (February 4, 2010), http://articles.mercola.com/sites/articles/archive/2010/02/04/stress-linked-to-cancer.aspx (accessed October 24, 2014).

2. "Panic and Anxiety Attacks and the Nervous System," Health-Science website, http://www.health-science.com/panic_and_anxiety_attacks_and_the_nervous_system.html (accessed September 29, 2014).

Rest

The time to relax is when you
don't have time for it.
—SYDNEY J. HARRIS

In his book, *Essentialism: The Disciplined Pursuit of Less*, Greg McKeown tells the story of Geoff, a go-getter with a huge heart to help others and who was really shaking the world up for the better. At 36, he was on the board of Kiva, he had been named "Entrepreneur of the Year" by Ernst and Young and a "Young Global Leader" by the World Economic Forum, he had co-founded a thriving impact investment fund, and he was the CEO of a microcredit organization that had touched the lives of more than 12 million poverty-stricken families all over the globe. If anybody were making a difference in the world, it was Geoff. A person would be hard pressed to find anyone who touched more lives than he did. He was constantly traveling all over the world and meeting with all kinds of different business leaders, non-governmental organization teams, and government representatives.

Between his schedule and jet lag, on average, Geoff slept between four and six hours a night. He kept promising himself he would catch up on some sleep when things settled down, but as the old saying goes, "Time waits for no man." There was always something new and more important that needed to be taken care of as soon as possible. So Geoff pushed on.

He began waking up in the middle of the night in stark panic. He would listen and look around, but there was no cause for alarm. These attacks gradually grew worse. His heart rate became erratic; and one by one, his organs began to malfunction and shut down. It became painful to stand, and he had to start putting his food in the blender because his digestive system refused to cooperate with him when he ate normally. His blood pressure dropped, and he'd black out if he stood up too fast. He was rushed to the emergency room twice, but he was sure he could just push through it.

He was wrong. After too many years of too little rest, he acknowledged it was time for a break. Faced with taking medications for the rest of his life or catching up on his rest, he agreed to take a month or two off, sure he could come back ready for anything after that. During the first month he slept fourteen hours a day and rested the remaining hours, often not even having the strength to get out of bed. At the end of two months, he knew he was still far from recovery. It would be two and a half years before he was able to go back to work. When he did finally get out again to attend a Young Global Leaders event in Tanzania, some of his friends who knew what he had been through asked what he had learned from the experience. Geoff told them he had paid a great price to learn a rather simple lesson: "Protect the asset."[1]

REST IS THE #1 KEY TO MANAGING STRESS AND LIFESTYLE DISEASES

While Geoff's experience is rather extreme, the message of what he experienced is a lesson to us. No matter how important what we are doing is, or how pressing the next crisis, we are no good to anyone if we are sick in bed or dead. Which do you think is better? Burned out and used up at 36? Or making steady, consistent impact on the world late into your 80s and 90s? To do the latter you have to have deep, regular, and consistent *rest*.

While few acknowledge it as such, stress is the true pandemic in the United States today. It is the most persistent risk factor hiding behind every chronic or lifestyle disease. According to British physician James Paget, "Fatigue (a direct result of stress) has a larger share in the promotion and transmission of disease than any other single condition you can name."[2] The real issue then is how do we balance times of stress with times of work, play, worship, and recovery? Balance is the key to rest.

The answer is not easy, but it is simple. For every period of stress, we need an equal or longer period of rest. While stress puts us on full alert, ramping up some body systems while virtually shutting everything else down, it is rest that allows us to adapt to the needs stress presses upon us. It is while we rest that we recover and build capacity so that we can do more the next time we face stress or strain. After all, we need stress to help us build muscle, strengthen our hearts, and expand our minds. Stress tests and stretches our limits; rest and recovery make it possible to handle that stress and then increase our capacity to handle it in the future.

WAKE-UP CALL

Time magazine reports that in 2012, Americans spent $32 billion on sleeping pills.

PHYSICAL REST

Of course, the best place to start getting rest is by getting the sleep we need. This generally means getting between seven and nine hours of sleep a night. Experts tell us the hours of sleep we get before midnight can be from two to four times more important than the hours we get after midnight. A good part of this is that melatonin production peaks at around 10 P.M.

According to alternative physician Joseph Pizzorno, ND, founder and President Emeritus of Bastyr University and author of *Total Wellness*:

> It's while we're sleeping that the body's regenerative processes are at work…. But in our society today, adequate sleep is becoming lost. If you look at the amount of sleep we get now compared to our grandparents, we are averaging almost two hours less sleep a night. And even when we are getting sleep, we aren't sleeping as deeply. We're sleeping later at night and bypassing the normal circadian rhythm that's created by nature."[3]

Many people struggle with insomnia—they can't get to sleep; or they fall asleep, but can't stay asleep. When that happens, most will turn to over-the-counter or prescription sleeping pills. These quick fixes bring with them a whole host of side effects, and don't address the real problems of sleep. Interrupted or impaired sleep stresses the whole body, weakens the immune system, accelerates tumor growth, causes your body to be hungry all the time, creates a fat-storing process in your digestive system, decreases your creativity and problem-solving ability, and weakens performance on all mental tasks throughout the day. Impaired sleep also increases stress-related disorders including heart disease, stomach ulcers, constipation, and mood disorders like depression.

Sleep deprivation prematurely ages you by interfering with production of human growth hormone. This important hormone that makes you both look and feel younger is usually secreted by your pituitary gland during periods of deep sleep as well as during periods of intense interval-type exercise.

So what are some of the problems interfering with healthy sleeping habits?

Problem #1: Sleeping on a Bad Mattress

I have a friend who sells mattresses for a living. He always says there are two things you shouldn't skimp on in your budget—shoes and mattresses. The reason? Because you are in one or the other of them all day long! When you are out of your shoes, you are on your mattress; and when you are up off your mattress, you are in your shoes! Wise advice from a simple man. Knowing this piece of information is not going to put more money in your budget, but it may give you the permission you need to realize that you are worth taking care of, and having a good quality mattress is an important part of that. Good quality pillows are also a must!

Problem #2: Sleeping with Lights On

Many don't realize that light of any kind disrupts your sleep patterns. Night lights, ambient light from electronic devices, bathroom lights, hall lights, daylight bleeding through the curtains at dawn—all these sources of light affect your sleep. Go to sleep and stay asleep in complete darkness. Get light blocking shades or curtains for your bedroom. If you need to get up at night, keep a small flashlight by your bed, then turn it out when you return. Don't keep computers, tablets, or phones on at night. The "blue light" rays they emit disrupt your natural sleep cycles.

Problem #3: Room Temperature

The optimal temperature for sleeping is between 60 and 68 degrees. Don't ever keep your bedroom above 70 degrees as it will cause you to sleep less deeply. Having a cool room mimics your body's natural drop in temperature during deep sleep cycles. If sleeping beside another person causes the temperature to go up too much, consider sleeping separately. Married couples did this for many hundreds of years, and there is no evidence that sleeping separately in and of itself damages the relationship.

Problem #4: EMFs

Electromagnetic fields are created from the use of electricity in your home. The only real way to check for electromagnetic fields is with a Gauss meter. But even without that tool, you can minimize the EMFs by following these suggestions:

- Don't run televisions, computers, tablets, or phones during the night.

- Shut them completely off to avoid electromagnetic "trash" from disrupting your pineal gland's production of melatonin and serotonin.

- If possible, move your bed away from touching the walls because most electrical wiring is buried there.

Problem #5: *Grand Central Bedroom*

To optimize sleep, don't watch television in bed. Also don't take your laptop or tablet to bed to work. By holding your bedtime and sleep time sacred, your body will receive the cue that when you lie down it is time to sleep…and nothing else.

While rest certainly means getting enough sleep, it also means making a cycle of rest in your life—taking at least one of the weekend days off to relax from work, emails, phone calls about work, and thoughts about work; and merely recreate. This doesn't mean lying on the couch watching sports, but doing something different from your regular weekday activities and enjoying some social time with friends and family. This also means creating a cycle of rest in each workday, perhaps including prayer and meditation, yoga, or exercise as ways to recharge your mind and "get the blood flowing."

INTERNAL REST

A less obvious but equally important way to give your body rest is to detoxify it, giving your systems rest from dealing with toxins that overtax your organs and systems. While we will talk at more length about this in the next chapter, for here let it suffice to say that reducing the toxins your body has to deal with on a daily basis gives your bodily systems the ability to run at normal levels rather than at constantly elevated levels. Eliminating toxins and increasing the intake of the right combinations of macro- and micronutrients as they are found in organic and whole foods allows your systems to handle more. When you live like this, your systems can run at a relatively relaxed, balanced pace, even when everything around you may be chaotic. This leaves every system of the body some room to ramp up when needed in order to give you the "superpowers" of the first stage of stress, but then to return to a level of homeostasis when the situation is over. This kind of rest allows for repair and recovery.

Homeostasis is the goal, and the only way to achieve that goal is to increase our neuroplasticity—our ability to adapt to and recover from stress, then return to a state of balance. Do you know why zebras never get ulcers? Robert Sapolsky, in his marvelous book, *Why Zebras Don't Get Sick,* tells us that zebras are at the bottom end of the food chain. Every other animal in their biosphere tries to eat them, and often succeeds. They have to be ready for an alert response all the time, because if they don't, they will be eaten for dinner! They are constantly scanning their environment for trouble. If they see or sense that trouble is brewing, they run away. If they don't run fast enough, all their problems are over. But if they do manage to escape, then they live to run the next day, and the next, and the next. And each and every time they stop running and they get to a place where they are safe, within a mere 90 seconds their nervous systems go back to normal! Zebras don't get ulcers because their systems are so neuroplastic that they adapt and respond immediately after the threat is over. The only time a zebra will get an ulcer is when it is locked in a zoo. It can't run away, so the stress never stops.

There is much in our environment that causes stress. Every day we are assaulted by stressors that we may not even be aware of because they have always been there. We call these stressors "pollution." Now when I say pollution, I'm not talking about some candy wrappers on the side of the road. I'm talking about substances that directly affect our nervous systems—noise pollution, air pollution, food pollution, and water pollution. Each day we are hearing, breathing, eating, and drinking toxic substances in tiny amounts. But as we age, those tiny amounts build and grow, doing unseen damage to our bodies.

Noise pollution seems like an antiquated idea because we have become so used to a high level of noise that we don't even consciously notice it. Because we aren't consciously aware of it, we don't spend time thinking about its harmful effects on our bodies. Noise pollution is mainly caused from machines and transportation (planes, trains, and cars), but the ever-present sounds of music, television, and news reports now pollute the inside of our buildings as much or more than machine noise pollutes the outside! High levels of constant noise affect our cardiovascular systems, and can cause constriction of the blood vessels, increased blood pressure, and increased stress that can lead to stroke or heart attack.[4] If you have ever said to your spouse or children, "Turn that TV down! My nerves are already frayed!" then you are experiencing the effects of noise pollution. Sometimes silence is the most restful state we can achieve.

Air pollution is also a stressor on our bodies. Thankfully our breathing is autonomic—which means we don't have to think about it every time we take a breath. But stop for a minute and think about what happens when you are startled or scared. You may gasp for breath, hold your breath, or begin to breathe in a shallow, nonproductive way. Our breath is our life. Air pollution is simply caused by waste. Whether it is the exhaust fumes from trucks and cars, secondhand smoke from tobacco, smoke from fires, or the gases that are emitted from factories during their normal course of production—it's all waste, and it is harmful to our health. One of the most prevalent but ignored sources of air pollution is right in our homes. "Pressboard" bookshelves and furniture emit toxic gases constantly right where we eat and sleep. These gases are proven hormone disruptors.

The respiratory system reacts to air pollution by sneezing and coughing. The cardiovascular system takes what has been breathed in and transports it to the blood, and eventually to the heart. Over time, air pollution can cause an inflammatory response in the heart, and even structural damage. Toxins that have been breathed in and have settled in our other organs can affect the efficiency of the whole cardiovascular system. Because these toxins damage arteries, our marvelous bodies adapt by sending fats (lipids) to the damaged arteries. Over time those fats choke and clog our arteries, and can lead to heart disease or death.[5]

Another often overlooked external stressor on our systems are the parabens present in almost every cosmetic and personal care product. A study published last year suggests that parabens from antiperspirants and other cosmetics appear to increase the risk of cancer, and most especially of breast cancer.[6] The research, which was also reviewed in an editorial published in the *Journal of Applied Toxicology*, looked at where breast tumors were appearing, and determined that higher concentrations of parabens were found in the upper quadrants of the breast area, where antiperspirants are usually applied.[7] The residues of parabens were found at concentrations up to *1 million times higher* than the estrogen levels naturally found in human breast tissue! These chemicals seem to be accumulating at alarmingly high concentrations, likely because of their widespread and persistent daily use. Previous research has shown that women absorb an estimated *five pounds* of chemicals a year from their daily makeup routines alone. Today, however, men are just as likely to get added toxins from shampoos, conditioners, aftershaves, and the like. The toxins present in these products enter our bodies through the epidermal layer (skin), and produce a buildup of chemicals known as the "total body burden."

So you see why we need to create habits of daily rest to give our bodies, minds, and hearts time to recuperate from the challenges behind us and around us, and to bolster ourselves for the ones ahead. This means finding a rhythm of grace in our lives so that we aren't chronically stressed and fatigued. It means building times of adaptation and recovery into our daily routines. It means getting quiet inside and out. And it means changing our habits of personal care, and perhaps our purchasing habits.

A RESTFUL LIFESTYLE

While McKeown's book, *Essentialism*, is a business book, not a health book, many of its principles reflect the value of rest and the necessity of keeping the important things in life from being eclipsed and run over by the urgent things in life. The basic premise of his book is that in order to live happier, healthier, and more productive lives, we should live by the maxim: "less, but better."

Many people are suffering unnecessarily with chronic illnesses brought on by lifestyle choices they didn't even know were harmful. In many cases, they followed the experts' advice and the government's standards of health; but now they are sicker than ever. Our culture has pushed them past their limits to keep up with some artificial standard of success; meanwhile, they were losing their most valuable asset—their health.

What McKeown shows in his book is that it is better to do a few things really well than a dozen things halfheartedly. To live as an essentialist means prioritizing our activities, maximizing our strengths, minimizing our weaknesses, and balancing the needs of our bodies, souls, careers, and families. We simply can't be all things to all people, and we need to learn to say "No!"

> *"Hey Doc, I know I'm supposed to sleep seven or eight hours a night, but who has time for that?"*
>
> The question is really, "Do you have time not to?" What if I told you that getting enough sleep every night would actually mean you got *more* done during the day than working more hours does? Charles A Czeisler, a sleep medicine professor at Harvard Medical School, likens sleep deprivation to drinking too much alcohol. In an article entitled, "Sleep Deficit: The Performance Killer," he wrote that just a week of getting only four or five hours of sleep a night "induces an impairment equivalent to a blood alcohol level of 0.1 percent,"[8] which means that person would not be legal to drive, let alone work!
>
> Not only that, but sleep deprivation generates a hormonal cascade, leaving you insulin resistant, craving sweets, and in fat-storing mode. Getting enough sleep will actually add time to your life in both the short and the long term.

From its inception, technology was supposed to simplify our lives and give us more free time. The problem has been, though, that it has had the opposite effect—instead of giving us more free time, technology makes us think we can do more things! As a result, we have created a "busyness bubble" around us fueled primarily by three things: smart phones, social media, and extreme consumerism. For the first time in the history of the world, we can be aware of what everyone else is doing, eating, reading, and buying—and for some reason, we seem to believe we should be keeping up with all that. After all, being super busy is code talk for being important and successful, isn't it?

Truly successful people are those who *choose* what they do, eat, read, and buy wisely and intentionally. They manage their eating, their exercise, and their overall health. They are mindful of why they are doing what they do, and it is not because they are trying to keep up with the proverbial Joneses. In order to live happier, healthier, more successful lives, we must pay attention to what we are doing. That means slowing down and recognizing the trade-offs for every activity and action Essentially, we can do one thing well, or two things less effectively and efficiently.

With this in mind, I would suggest creating some "technology-free" times in your day, particularly when you are at home. Turning off the television and instead reading or playing games the last hour before bedtime is not going to hurt anyone in your home. Having a sit-down dinner together three or four times a week would be a change for most families, but you would be surprised how much better your relationship with your kids will be if you do that! Research suggests that families who eat dinner together three or more times a week have children who are less likely to be overweight, will eat more healthy food, have less delinquency, are less likely to abuse alcohol or drugs, show greater academic achievement, exhibit healthier psychological well-being, and have more positive family interactions.[9] All of this adds up to more happiness and less stress!

Another way to create a restful lifestyle is to build free time into your family's schedule. Kids don't need to participate in more than one sport or activity a season, nor must they always be occupied. There is nothing wrong with having your kids exploring things they can do on their own while at home with you.

Orderliness is yet another way to create a restful lifestyle. Don't buy new clothes without taking some time to go through the closet and drawers to get rid of some of the things that no longer fit or never get worn. Regularly go through your house to give away things that you don't use but that might be a blessing to others. It can be as important to keep a clutter-free living space as it is to have a clutter-free mind! An orderly environment will cause less stress than a chaotic environment.

You can't live by the maxim "less but better" without making choices, but those choices help you stay in control of your life and your future. Forcing yourself to make the hard choices is the best way to remember what is truly important. If you don't make value choices about your time, energy, and money, then you will soon be out of all three of them!

Caring for Your Health Is Never for the Back Burner

It's really odd how often we take our health for granted. In no other important area of our lives would we wait until a problem rears its ugly head to create a management plan. Not in our finances, not in our romantic relationships, not in our childrearing! Why then would we think it would work with our health? Should you wait until you come home one night to find all of your bags packed sitting at the end of the front walk before you nurture your marriage? Do you wait until the bill collectors are calling before you pay your bills? Do you wait until your credit card is declined before you pay attention to its balance?

Yet this is exactly what we do with our health. For some reason we believe we can eat whatever we want, never work out, think that whatever tastes good is good for us, and assume that genetics and getting older are the cause of all of our health issues because that is what everyone else is telling us. No, that doesn't work. What we need is the courage and discipline to create lifestyles that are characterized by peace and restfulness, not stress and restlessness!

NOTES

1. Greg McKeown, *Essentialism: The Disciplined Pursuit of Less* (New York: Crown Business, 2014), 91-94.

2. Elmer A. Josephson, *God's Key to Health and Happiness* (Old Tappan, NJ: Power Books, 1962), 163.

3. Larry Trivieri, "Understanding Your Body's Healing Systems: An Interview with Joseph Pizzorno, N. D." *The Healthy Edge Letter* Vol. 1, no. 5 (December 1998), 8.

4. "Road Noise Link to Blood Pressure," BBC News, September 10, 2009, http://news.bbc.co.uk/2/hi/health/8247217.stm.

5. "Cardiovascular Effects of Air Pollution," Health Canada, October 18, 2013, accessed December 16, 2014, http://www.hc-sc.gc.ca/ewh-semt/air/out-ext/health-sante/cardio-eng.php.

6. L. Barr et al., "Measurement of Paraben Concentrations in Human Breast Tissue at Serial Locations across the Breast from Axilla to Sternum," *Journal of Applied Toxicology* 32, no. 3 (2012): 219-232, doi:10.1002/jat.1786.

7. Philip W. Harvey and David J. Everett, "Parabens Detection in Different Zones of the Human Breast: Consideration of Source and Implications of Findings," *Journal of Applied Toxicology* 32, no. 5 (2012): 305-309, doi:10.1002/jat.2743.

8. Charles A. Czeisler, "Sleep Deficit: The Performance Killer," interview by Bronwyn Fryer, *Harvard Business Review* (Oct 2006), http://hbr.org/2006/10/sleep-deficit-the-performance-killer (accessed September 22, 2014).

9. Eliza Cook and Rachel Dunifon, "Do Family Meals Really Make a Difference?" Cornell University, College of Human Ecology, http://www.human.cornell.edu/pam/outreach/upload/Family -Mealtimes-2.pdf (accessed October 30, 2014).

Step Six

Detox

The wealth and privilege associated with
modern America have come at a terrible price
to our overall health. We have created a diet
and lifestyle that is so toxic that we've become
toxic, too—and it is killing us. Our air is toxic;
our water is polluted; our food is depleted
of nutrients and packed with poisonous
chemicals and hormones; viruses and unhealthy
bacteria are rampant. Not only that, but our
minds and hearts often get polluted also.
—DON COLBERT, MD

Natalie started working in our office in January of 2012, but she came in with more health issues than some of our patients. For generations, the women in Natalie's family had a history of endometriosis (trouble with the lining of the uterus) and hysterectomies by the age of 30. When she began having a number of health issues related to heavy and erratic menstrual cycles in her early 20s, she couldn't help but wonder if she were headed for the same fate.

She hit a wall when one of her cycles lasted 41 days and only ended when she took a prescription to stop it. All she wanted to do was sleep, but she never felt safe being far away from a bathroom because of the heavy bleeding.

She'd been to several doctors already, but she continued to try new ones hoping that one of them would have a solution. Finally an ob-gyn admitted her to the hospital after seeing her low hemoglobin levels. She spent the next two days in the hospital, receiving two blood transfusions. They prescribed birth-control pills, and as a result, she didn't have a period for the next three months. Still not knowing what was wrong, she continued to try to find a physician who would know how to solve this condition, not merely treat the symptoms.

Then one day, out of the blue, she began to experience painful cramps and nausea about 1:00 in the afternoon. This continued for the next six hours. She felt clammy, was short of breath, and experienced the worst stomach pain of her entire life. She finally decided to go to the hospital, and took some Advil right before she left hoping it would help. When she got to the emergency room, she was told there would be a three-hour wait before she could be seen. After about an hour, the pain decreased slightly. In the end, the doctors didn't know what to do differently, so they simply sent her home.

The next day when she was going to the bathroom, a large chunk of tissue came out. She naturally panicked and called her doctor. She took a picture of the tissue and sent it to him. She thought she had just shed her uterus all in one piece. But when her doctor got a look at it, he told her the tissue was part of a cyst she would need to have surgically removed. The next day they performed a hysteroscopy and removed a five-centimeter cyst. Thankfully the biopsy showed it was benign. Her doctor put her on progesterone, but her cycles came back stronger and heavier than before, lasting anywhere from 30-50 days.

It was soon after that Natalie started working with us and she began absorbing all the information we were teaching to our patients. In a matter of weeks she had completely transformed her diet. This helped a little, but not completely. Then, after a few months with us, we had a patient who came in with symptoms very similar to Natalie's. We eventually linked these symptoms back to an improperly done root canal. Soon after, Natalie remembered that she had had a root canal as well about six years earlier. We recommended that she immediately go to a holistic dentist to have it checked out. Sure enough, there was an infection in her mouth from the root canal and the dentist suggested the tooth be removed as soon as possible.

The day she went in for the extraction, Natalie was on the 30th day of her cycle. Eight days after the tooth was removed, her cycle stopped on its own, which was the first time that had happened without medical intervention in years. Shortly after that she had her first normal cycle since the age of fourteen.

During this entire time, Natalie had not, of course, been able to conceive. After the tooth was removed her body healed itself with the help of excellent nutrition, improved neuroplasticity, and a correct exercise program. As a result, Natalie gave birth to a healthy baby girl, Brooklyn Rain, on August 7, 2014.

I've included Natalie's story for a couple of reasons. First, I want you to see the incredible effects toxic chemical stress can have on our bodies, even from infections we don't realize are there. Secondly, I want you to see how easily we can be fooled when we are looking at the wrong indicators. None of Natalie's doctors were looking for the cause of the toxic stress. Each doctor was merely trying to treat her symptoms. A third reason is that I want you to see how toxic stress can hide, literally right under our noses, and we won't find it unless we are looking in the right place. In this case, as in so many others, adopting the proper paradigm or "set of glasses" makes all the difference in the world.

UNDERSTANDING TOXIC STRESS

We have no idea how many toxins we absorb into our bodies on a day-to-day basis, and we know even less how those chemicals affect our health. In a 2006 article for *National Geographic*, reporter David Ewing Duncan asked that very question: Just how many chemicals do normal human beings have in their bodies without even realizing it? The answer shocked him. Using himself as a human guinea pig, he allowed himself to be tested for 320 different chemical substances. His body showed traces of at least 165 of them. Some of his levels were relatively low, however, others were alarmingly high—higher than the normal level for factory workers who spend every day working in the presence of those same chemicals.[1] Mr. Duncan isn't a factory worker, though, he's a journalist, and not one who spends any of his time in chemical or manufacturing plants. According to the article, his body tested positive for:

> ...Older chemicals that [he] might have been exposed to decades ago, such as DDT and PCBs; pollutants like lead, mercury, and dioxins; newer pesticides and plastic ingredients; and the near-miraculous compounds

that lurk just beneath the surface of modern life, making shampoos fragrant, pans nonstick, and fabrics water-resistant and fire-safe.[2]

While more research will need to be done in order to determine just how such chemicals affect us, it's not surprising that each of them adds a degree of toxic stress to our bodies. The more toxic chemical load present in any human, the greater the degree of health complications that will be present.

Take **lead** for example. In 1971 the U.S. Surgeon General announced that any level of lead below 40 micrograms per deciliter of blood was safe. Now we know that even a trace of lead can be detrimental, especially in children where it has been shown to cause neurological damage and reduced IQs. It is very possible that the levels of **arsenic** in our orange juice and rice, the levels of **mercury** in our fish, and the levels of **fluoride** and **chloride** in our water, that are now deemed safe, may one day be determined by our government to be extremely dangerous. It wouldn't be the first time they were wrong.

Our bodies are stressed, and we don't know it. In the beginning our bodies try to keep up, recover, compensate and do what they can to survive. Once these coping strategies get overwhelmed, the problems that have been flying below the radar get expressed as symptoms that arise. Television commercials and marketing campaigns advise us to take something to suppress the symptoms. Birth control for heavy bleeding, Advil for pain, Pepcid for reflux. When we suppress those symptoms, it makes it that much harder to find the real culprit. For instance, we are faced each day with endocrine-disrupting chemicals that our grandparents never had to face. The **BPA** found in food cans, water bottles, and cell phone protectors disrupts our hormonal balance adding to estrogen overload. BPA is even found in the coating on every store receipt that you handle! This dangerous chemical affects every system in the body. It can lead to prostate or breast cancer, uterine fibroids, weight gain, cardiovascular disease, diabetes, early onset of puberty, and a whole host of other problems.

Synthetic estrogen is found in all oral birth control pills. It has been identified as a major cause of cancers in women. We are all exposed to this toxin as millions of these pills are flushed into the water supply every year. As we drink our tap water, we are being exposed to far too much estrogen. This again disrupts our normal hormonal balance.

Fire retardants that coat our furniture, clothing, and bedding contain a dangerous form of **bromine** that interferes with normal thyroid function. The thyroid is in charge of metabolism and energy and needs iodine to function properly. Because bromine is in the same family as iodine, it competes for dominance in the thyroid gland. It often wins, creating an underactive thyroid. So doctors prescribe thyroid medication, but never address *why* the thyroid is struggling in the first place.

The **fluoride** and **chloride** in our drinking water are also in the same family as iodine, and as you may have guessed, they also compete for dominance in the thyroid gland. Between bromine (found in fire retardants and in many soft drinks) and the fluoride and perchlorate (chlorine) in our water, the poor iodine molecules lose out—and ultimately so does our health! Low thyroid function causes weight gain, fatigue, and depression. White flour is bleached that unnatural white color by using chlorine gas, so by all means avoid white flour!

Phthalates are found in plastics—plastic bags, plastic cups, plastic storage containers, plastic water bottles, anything plastic.

They add flexibility and resilience to plastic, but they are toxic! Chronic exposure to phthalates has been linked to obesity, low sperm count, diabetes, and thyroid conditions. Because of this, we encourage everyone to store as much as they can in glass instead of plastic; and by all means, don't heat your food in plastic containers in a microwave oven! This is a health disaster waiting to happen.

Arsenic is found beneath the earth's crust, but it can leach into the water supply whenever that crust is disrupted through construction, excavation, or mining. Exposure to arsenic can result in insulin resistance, immune system suppression, slowed cognitive development, cardiovascular damage, and weight gain/loss. The best way to protect against arsenic is to install a water filter, one that specifically contains the ability to remove arsenic. Trace amounts of arsenic are also present in processed orange juice. Avoid bottled juices whenever possible, and opt for freshly juiced, organic fruits and vegetables.

PFCs (perfluorinated chemicals) are found in non-stick cookware. If you own this type of cookware, replace it as soon as you can. When heated, PFCs leach into your food. This toxin is also used to coat the insides of bags of microwave popcorn. If you eat microwaved popcorn, you should stop immediately. Once PFCs start to accumulate in your body, they can cause infertility, ineffective sperm, heart disease, thyroid disease, high cholesterol, and low birth weight in babies. A recent study confirmed PFCs, especially **PFOA** and **PFHxS**, negatively affect thyroid hormone levels. A deep and thorough cleansing may be helpful for removing built-up levels of PFCs in the body.

Mercury is toxic and dangerous to pregnant women and the babies they carry. It's known to affect women in particular as it will bind with a hormone essential to menstruation and ovulation.

Mercury also attacks the pancreas, thereby affecting insulin production. This action may lead to diabetes; however, research is unclear on this topic. Reducing seafood consumption may be one of the best solutions to reducing mercury intake; unfortunately, fish is no longer the only concern. Immunizations often contain mercury as a carrier. Many parents choose not to immunize their children because they believe that exposure to childhood diseases is far less dangerous than exposure to a known neurotoxin. The new CFL lightbulbs contain dangerous levels of mercury. In fact, if one of these lightbulbs break, it's recommended you evacuate the area to prevent exposure.

Aluminum is a toxin that finds its way quickly to the human brain where it is stored. The use of aluminum cookware has been implicated in human toxicity, as has the use of antiperspirants and over-the-counter heartburn and indigestion remedies. Professor Chris Exley from Keeley University, UK is an expert in the field of research relating to Alzheimer's disease. He is adamant that at some point in time, the accumulation of aluminum in the brain will achieve a toxic threshold and a specific neuron or area of the brain will stop coping with the presence of aluminum and will start reacting to its presence. If the same brain tissue is also suffering other insults or another ongoing degenerative condition, then the additional response to aluminum will make worse these effects. So aluminum may cause other conditions to be more aggressive or to have an earlier onset. These occurrences have already been shown in Alzheimer's disease related to environmental and occupational exposure to aluminum.

Acrylamides are found in fried foods like French fries and potato chips. They are also present whenever you "char" meat on a grill, or even in a pan on the stove. They are present in cigarettes. Avoid fried foods, cigarettes, and charred meat products whenever possible as acrylamides build up in your body and cause serious damage.

Genetically modified foods are all around us, and big agribusiness is pushing for more! The Monsanto Company is leading the way to influence lawmakers and consumers alike to accept genetically modified corn, soybeans, potatoes, and grains, even though GMOs have been shown to cause immune system, brain, and liver damage.

The number-one source of calories taken in by Americans today is from **high fructose corn syrup**. Starting in the 1970s, processed food manufacturers began using this damaging chemical instead of sucrose or table sweetener. Why did they do this? Because it was cheaper, and it produced a sweeter product. The generations of children who grew up with sweeter food crave that same level of satisfaction now that they are adults. This is one reason for the preponderance of obesity in our country today. Not only does high fructose corn syrup cause weight gain and metabolic problems, it also increases triglyceride levels and raises "bad" (LDL) cholesterol. Around 100 years ago the average American consumed a mere 15 grams of fructose a day, primarily in the form of fruit. One hundred years later, one-fourth of Americans are consuming more than 135 grams per day, largely in the form of soda. At 15 grams a day, fructose is harmless. However, at nearly ten times that amount it becomes a major cause of obesity and nearly all chronic degenerative disease.

So what did many of these overweight adults turn to? Diet sodas and "diet" foods filled with toxic **artificial sweeteners**. Now it seemed that we could have all the satisfaction with none of the guilt! The only problem is that artificial sweeteners can cause convulsions and make you crave more sweets. They can also cause weight gain and lead to diabetes. They produce toxins in the stomach when broken down by the body. **Aspartame**, the most commonly consumed artificial sweetener in America, is used in over 6,000 products worldwide despite its having been linked to a host of health problems including brain tumors and brain cancer, lymphomas, Leukemia and other blood cancers, as well as breast and prostate cancer. It is an "excitotoxin," and all excitotoxins increase the growth of cancer cells. This is a relatively easy one to eliminate from your life. Avoid *any* artificial sweeteners.

Another of the biggest stressors to our bodies in America today is a dangerous chemical that has been banned in many countries across Europe—**glycophosphate**. You have probably used this powerful defoliant to control the weeds in your yard. Known by the commercial trade name *Roundup*, glycophosphate is toxic, and it is used in the production and harvest of most of our foods. Many people think they are eating healthfully when they buy apples, grapes, or strawberries from the store. But unless these fruits are organic or verified to be pesticide-free, they could be a major cancer risk. The Environmental Working Group (EWG) found that up to 98 percent of all conventional produce, and particularly the type found on its "dirty" fruits list, is contaminated with cancer-causing pesticides.

Are you beginning to see how much stress is put on our bodies from toxic chemicals every single day? According to the Center for Disease Control (CDC), it is estimated that over 80 percent of all illnesses have environmental and lifestyle causes. Not only can what we are exposed to make us ill, but the accumulation of toxins over the years can wreak havoc with our health. The more toxic our bodies are, the more our interior environment is stressed. Numerous diseases like arthritis, allergies, autoimmune diseases, and digestive dysfunction are all caused by an immune system that is so overloaded it begins to attack indiscriminately, striking at healthy cells as well as foreign pathogens.

While we have yet to determine the exact effects of all of these chemicals on our systems, it is safe to say that most of them weren't around 100 years ago, and that the epidemic levels of cancer and other stress-related diseases we are seeing today were much lower back then as well. Over 69 million Americans live in large cities and areas that regularly exceed smog standards.[3] Most tap water contains over 700 chemicals, sometimes including high concentrations of lead.[4] Roughly 3,000 chemicals have been added to our food supply, and we are daily exposed to as many as 10,000 chemicals in the form of solvents, emulsifiers, and preservatives, many of which can remain in the body for years. According to Phyllis Saifer, MD, in her book *Detox*, "It is estimated that the average American ingests one gallon of food additives yearly."[5] Do we really think we can be taking all of this into our bodies without negatively affecting our health?

DETOXIFYING IS NOT A ONE-AND-DONE FIX

There is no way to avoid getting some toxins in our systems in varying quantities. The good news is that our bodies routinely handle a lot of the cleansing and detoxification all on their own. Several key organs in the body have specific detoxifying responsibilities, like the liver, the kidneys, the lungs, the colon, and even our skin, which loves to sweat things out that our body doesn't want. The lymphatic system, which is a little like the body's version of a sewage system, pulls refuse from every cell in our body and takes it away for disposal. This very fact means that the best way to detoxify is to give our bodies as much rest as we can from toxins so that our systems can "clean house" for themselves.

"Hey Doc, I don't really have the money or time to do an expensive detox program or juice fast. Are there simple, affordable ways to detoxify my body?"

Yes! One simple way is to take a bath with half cup of baking soda, two cups of Epsom salts, two tablespoons of coconut oil, and a few drops of lavender essential oil. This will not only serve as a whole body detox (remember the skin is the largest organ of the human body), but the magnesium and lavender will calm you down and give you a great night's sleep!

Here are six common-sense habits that will encourage and support the body's natural detoxification systems:

1. Make whole organic foods, living nutrients, and super foods the center of your diet. Make sure you are getting as much nutrition as you can through the foods you eat.

Consuming natural, organic, unprocessed, and properly prepared foods is crucial. It is better to eat organic fruits, vegetables, meats, and dairy, because these aren't loaded down with commercial pesticides, fungicides, antibiotics, and preservatives. In addition, after repeated testing, organic produce and proteins have been shown to be more nutritious than their nonorganic counterparts.

WHAT QUALIFIES AS *ORGANIC*?

According to the USDA:

"Organic food is produced by farmers who emphasize the use of renewable resources and the conservation of soil and water to enhance environmental quality for future generations. Organic meat, poultry, eggs, and dairy products come from animals that are given no antibiotics or growth hormones. Organic food is produced without using most conventional pesticides; fertilizers made with synthetic ingredients or sewage sludge; bioengineering; or ionizing radiation. Before a product can be labeled "organic," a government-approved certifier inspects the farm where the food is grown to make sure the farmer is following all the rules necessary to meet USDA organic standards. Companies that handle or process organic food before it gets to your local supermarket or restaurant must be certified, too."[6]

2. Practice advanced hygiene.

According to the *Merriam-Webster Dictionary, hygiene* means, "conditions or practices (as of cleanliness) conducive to health." Certainly this means regular bathing, but beyond that it also means to be careful of what you are putting on your skin, in your hair, and into your mouth. Creams, dyes, shampoos, soaps, cosmetics, deodorant, mouthwash, toothpaste—these items all carry toxic ingredients unless they are labeled otherwise. We need to be mindful of the five ways germs and viruses and chemical toxins enter the body: through the skin on our hands as well as through the mouth, nose, ears, and eyes.

3. Condition your body regularly with exercise, stretching, and body therapies.

Exercise and stretching facilitates detoxification by increasing the oxygen in your cells and expelling gaseous wastes as well as massaging or shaking the lymphatic system, which collects waste from the body to remove it. Rebounding on a trampoline, walking, or other cardio and stretching workouts are great for helping several systems of the body cleanse themselves.

4. Reduce toxins in your environment.

From the materials that your home and workplace were constructed with, to the products used to clean them, toxic chemicals surround you. This isn't something that should frighten you, but you do want to be aware of it and look for cleaners that are made of natural products. This is especially important to consider when cleaning the surfaces where you prepare food and eat.

5. Avoid toxic emotions.

We have enough problems every day without hanging on to grudges, past hurts, disappointments, or other emotional dead weight. Life can be full of barbs and slights, but we still have the power to choose our reactions. What good will holding a grudge do you anyway? Choose gratitude and forgiveness instead. As it has been said, "Refusing to forgive is like drinking poison and expecting the other person to die."

6. Live a contemplative and purposeful life.

We contemplate because deep, logical thought is God's gift to man. He gave this to no other creature. When we think deeply and contemplate the meaning of our lives—what we are to accomplish while we are here and how we are going to enrich the lives of others along the way, we develop purpose. A purposeful life is a life worth living. Self-help books will generally tell us to look to our desires and our dreams for our purpose, but the richest, healthiest, and most successful individuals in history have been that way because they realized, accepted, and lived God's purpose for them. Once you reclaim your health and vitality, what mission will you be on? How will you use this newfound energy to bless our broken world?

FASTING

Your body was made to cleanse itself daily, but if you are eating unhealthy foods and/or "grazing" around the clock, then your digestive system never really has the time to rest and recover as other systems do. Fasting—even for short amounts of time each day—gives your body a chance to cleanse and heal itself. Fasting can also help break addictions to junk food, drinking, smoking, television, or any number of habits or addictions that you may want to be free of. It supports the body's detoxification organs and systems and promotes healthy weight loss, if done correctly. Fasting also raises energy levels; improves memory, focus, and concentration; aids in stress relief; and encourages sounder sleep. It improves cardiovascular health; promotes healthy digestion and elimination; improves inflammation response, joint comfort, and hormonal balance; makes your skin healthier and clearer; and helps boost immune function.[7] Considering all of those benefits, it makes sense to be hungry on purpose every once and a while.

Now I know fasting probably doesn't sound like a whole lot of fun, but fasting doesn't just mean going without food for days on end. This would not be practical for most of us. But regular times of fasting for 24 or 48 hours can be extremely helpful in regaining discipline in your life while at the same time resting your body's systems. Food isn't the only thing that you can fast. If you have an addictive habit like watching too much TV, spending too much time surfing the Internet, keeping up with social media, smoking, chewing gum, or complaining; declaring a time of "fasting" from those activities can be a great way to break their power over you. Another added benefit is that fasting will likely point out some of the cues that trigger those habits in the first place so that you can then respond differently to those cues.

As far as fasting for health reasons, you don't have to cut out all foods for your fast to be effective. In fact, going on a partial fast—like a juice fast, a "Daniel fast,"[8] a sugar fast, a gluten fast, or some combination of any of those—is basically what health practitioners call an "elimination" diet. The idea behind an elimination diet is to take out the things that may be negatively affecting your health and only eat what is known to be safe. J.J. Virgin's *The Virgin Diet* is based on eliminating the seven foods that we as human beings most often show an intolerance for: 1) sugar and artificial sweeteners, 2) gluten, 3) dairy, 4) soy, 5) corn, 6) peanuts, and 7) eggs. She then encourages adding them back into your diet one at a time to see what effect they have on you. Many are surprised to discover that they experience unpleasant side effects after eliminating, then reintroducing problem foods. This type of fast is great for determining what foods you should avoid.

WAKE-UP CALL

An eight-ounce glass of orange juice (even fresh-squeezed) has eight teaspoons of sugar as compared with ten in an eight-ounce can of soda.

The Daniel fast is a perfect fit for many people. It is based on the story of Daniel from the Bible. Daniel and three of his friends refused to eat from the king's banquet table to honor their religious food traditions, choosing instead only "pulse" (basically beans or vegetables) and water for ten days. According to the book of Daniel:

> At the end of ten days it was seen that they were better in appearance and fatter in flesh than all the youths who ate the king's food. So the steward took away their food and the wine they were to drink, and gave them vegetables.[9]

So history records that Daniel and his friends were actually healthier after those ten days than all of the other students in the king's palace who ate the delicacies and other dishes made by the king's chefs. I'm not sure if Daniel was the first vegetarian or not, but he is certainly the first one in recorded history to have adopted this plan by choice and have it recognized as healthier than what others were eating at the time.

DID YOU KNOW?

Fasting extends your lifespan and protects against disease. It also increases insulin sensitivity (shutting off your hunger more quickly), makes mitochondrial energy distribution more efficient, and reduces oxidative stress while increasing our capacity to resist stress and aging.

Another form of fasting that is beneficial is known as *intermittent fasting*. Intermittent fasting is a daily fast of 16 to 18 hours, or roughly half of our normal waking hours. Most people who do this keep a schedule where they only eat between 11 am and 7 pm, or a commensurate span of time. While this contradicts the old saying, "breakfast is the most important meal of the day," I think you would be surprised by the benefits of starting your day with "first meal" at 11 o'clock instead.

One reason for intermittent fasting is that it takes six to eight hours for our systems to metabolize our glycogen stores from the food we just ate. When we burn through those stores, our bodies burn fat to create energy instead. If we eat every four to six hours, our bodies never need to burn fat for fuel, so we hang on to the fat we don't want. Calorie restriction has been shown to increase the lifespan of certain animals by as much as 50 percent. Recent studies, however have shown that intermittent fasting without strict calorie restriction may be as effective as calorie restriction in increasing lifespan.

Biologist Satchidananda Panda and colleagues at Salk's Regulatory Biology Laboratory published one of the most significant studies in the effects of intermittent fasting in 2012. They fed two groups of mice high-fat, high-calorie diets. They allowed the first group to have access to food 24 hours a day, while the second group was allowed access only during their most active eight hours; and then they fasted the rest of the time. Both groups consumed the same number of calories during each 24-hour period. However, the results for each group were dramatically different. Those with 24-7 access to food grew obese and showed evidence of high cholesterol, high blood sugar, fatty liver disease, and metabolic problems. Those that fasted 16 hours a day but still ate the same amount of calories remained lean and did not develop any of these same health issues. They concluded, "[Intermittent fasting] is a non-pharmacological strategy against obesity and associated diseases."[10] Other studies have shown that intermittent fasting has other benefits as well. One such benefit is in switching your body from its growth and aging mode to its repair mode. Another benefit is that it lowers the risk of diabetes and cancer. This discipline of intermittent fasting also triggers the production of human growth hormone (HGH) in men, reducing oxidative stress and benefitting the brain, mental well-being, and clarity of thought.[11]

All of this to say that you can be creative with how you fast. Consider a "fast" of things you shouldn't put into your system or a nutrition protocol that focuses on only eating real foods that are organic. The main idea is to reduce the body's toxic load and increase its vital nutrients. Find things that you like, find the foods that will help with your cravings and keep your hunger in check, and be creative. After all, healthy eating should be fun; otherwise, who would want to do it?

CREATING A NEW MEDICAL HISTORY FOR YOUR FAMILY

Recently Dr. Oz cited a number of studies saying that my city, Knoxville, Tennessee, is the unhealthiest city in America. This despite the fact that it has more hospitals per capita than anywhere else in the country. According to a Blue Cross/Blue Shield report from just a few years ago, the average patient in this city has a prescription load of 18.3 pills *per day*.

Considering this, let me ask: If good healthcare and getting the right medications are the key to better health, wouldn't Knoxville be the *healthiest* city in America rather than the *unhealthiest*? I mean, if Knoxville has more hospitals per person than anywhere else and more medications per person than anywhere else, why is it the unhealthiest city in America? Just how does that work? That would mean there are remote places in the frozen tundra of Alaska that are healthier than Knoxville! There are ghettos in New York, Los Angeles, Chicago, and Detroit that are healthier than Knoxville. There are places in the middle of the desert in Nevada where the few families who live there have to drive more than 50 miles to get to the nearest hospital. And still they are healthier than people living within a couple of blocks of a hospital in Knoxville. Despite all of our resources, Knoxville is still the unhealthiest city in America. If better access to healthcare is the answer, then how can that be?

WAKE-UP CALL

From 1992-2002, prescriptions for opiates rose 400 percent.

America as a nation consumes 72 percent of the world's supply of drugs.

NOTES

1. David Ewing Duncan, "Toxic People," *National Geographic* magazine (Oct. 2006), http://ngm.nationalgeographic.com/2006/10/toxic-people/duncan-text/1 (accessed: September 18, 2014).

2. Ibid., 2.

3. Environmental Protection Agency, "EPA Data Show Steady Progress in Cleaning Nation's Air," *Environmental News* (October 1992), as reported in: "Did You Know." *Our Toxic Times* Vol. 3 no. 12 (December 1992), 5.

4. Environmental Protection Agency, "130 Cities Exceed Lead Levels for Drinking Water," *Environmental News* (October 1992).

5. Phyllis Saifer, MD, *Detox* (Los Angeles: Jeremy P. Tarcher, 1984), 42.

6. "National Organic Movement," USDA website, http://www.ams .usda.gov/AMSv1.0/ams.fetchTemplateData.do?template =TemplateN&leftNav=NationalOrganicProgram&page =NOPGoingOrganic&description=Going+Organic (accessed September 24, 2014).

7. Jordan Rubin, *The Maker's Diet Revolution* (Shippensburg, PA: Destiny Image Publishers, Inc., 2013), 34-35.

8. There are several books out with the terms "Daniel fast" or "Daniel plan" in their titles. My personal favorite, though, is *The Maker's Diet* or *The Maker's Diet Revolution* by my good friend Jordan Rubin. I would highly recommend either of those. Rick Warren's *The Daniel Plan* is also a good resource.

9. Daniel 1:15-16.

10. Megumi Hatori, Christopher Vollmers, Amir Zarrinpar, Luciano DiTacchio, Eric A. Bushong, Shubhroz Gill, Mathias Leblanc, Amandine Chaix, Matthew Joens, James A.J. Fitzpatrick, Mark H. Ellisman, Satchidananda Panda, "Time-Restricted Feeding without Reducing Caloric Intake Prevents Metabolic Diseases in Mice Fed a High-Fat Diet," *Cell Metabolism*, vol. 15, no. 6 (June 6, 2012), 848-860, http://www.sciencedirect.com/science/article/pii/ S1550413112001891 (accessed October 28, 2014).

11. Joseph Mercola, MD, "How Intermittent Fasting Stacks Up Among Obesity-Related Myths, Assumptions, and Evidence-Backed Facts," *Peak Fitness* (March 1, 2013), http://fitness.mercola .com/sites/fitness/archive/2013/03/01/daily-intermittent-fasting .aspx (accessed: October 28, 2014).

Step Seven

Nourishment

You can pay the farmer now, or the doctor later.

—JORDAN RUBIN

Elizabeth was another person who joined one of our "Get Well" programs after attending a seminar I facilitated with Jordan Rubin. She'd read *The Maker's Diet* years before, but never acted on it. This time, though, she and her husband were ready to eat more healthfully. She found the plan easy to follow; and after the initial three days her energy had increased, her skin glowed, and she'd already lost weight.

By the end of the full two weeks, she felt so much better she decided she would stay with the program. The plan was easy to follow, and the foods left her satisfied. She felt better than she had in years! Because she had a tendency to overeat, she was worried about not counting calories. Counting calories had always been her "safety zone." What she found, however, was that her cravings and desire to eat more than she needed were never anything she couldn't handle. All of that, and in the two weeks she lost 17 pounds!

The fact of the matter is, good nutrition isn't rocket science. As you are probably starting to realize by this point, the key principle is to eat real food in as natural and organic a state as possible. Once you get into the program, you start to get the hang of the meal planning pretty quickly, and it can have amazing results on both your health and your waistline. Elizabeth didn't have amazing healing happen in her body because her health had not yet broken down. She wasn't in need of radical repair, but she saw that impending iceberg and corrected the course of her life. In effect, Elizabeth changed her own medical history.

#1) EAT REAL FOOD

I believe we are truly in the midst of a food revolution. Books like Michael Moss's *Salt Sugar Fat* and documentaries like *Supersize Me*, *Forks over Knives*, and *Fed Up* are shedding light on what our food industry has become. They are exposing how manufacturers are manipulating our taste buds for their own profits to the detriment of our health, and why obesity has grown to such a point that in most of the world it is a greater health risk than hunger or poverty.

More and more information is available every day to help consumers make better choices as to what they buy and what they eliminate. Getting rid of foods that are not only low in nutrition and encourage overeating, but are also filled with toxins that stress our bodily systems and cause them to break down is easier than you think.

WAKE-UP CALL

According to the World Health Organization (WHO), 65 percent of the world's population live in countries where obesity kills more people than being underweight.[1]

Though we don't have room here to go into all of the different great-tasting recipes that are possible with real food, you can get many of them at our monthly Unhealthy Anonymous meetings. They are also available on our website at www.unhealthyanonymous.com, and we are in the process of creating a comprehensive cookbook as a companion resource. Here are some of the basics for choosing *real* foods:

- Vegetables should become the foundation of your new food pyramid, replacing the traditional breads, cereals, rice, and pastas that all come from grains. The more living your vegetables and fruits are when you eat them, the better.

- Avoid sugar and gluten as much as possible, especially in beverages and white breads. These are toxins and are literally killing America. Alcohol and caffeine should also be avoided as much as possible. Beer, wine, and many liquors contain sugars and gluten.

- Avoid *all* processed foods. As author and food expert Michael Pollan puts it: "If it's a plant, eat it. If it was made in a plant, don't."

- Start reading labels. Here, again, the rule for purchasing is pretty simple: *if there is an ingredient on the label you can't pronounce, don't buy it.*

- Avoid "diet," "low-fat," or "fat-free" products. "Diet" usually means they have replaced sugar with an artificial sweetener, and removed fats that your body actually needs.

- Just because it says "organic," "gluten-free," "whole," "natural," or "sugar-free" doesn't mean that it's healthy for you. In fact, there is no standard for what can be labeled "natural"—anyone can use that term.

- Canned or packaged real foods normally have a simple list of ingredients (usually five or fewer), all of which are able to be recognized as foods and not as chemicals or sugars.

- Also make sure to watch the carbohydrates! Now that manufacturers are increasing the sugar, fat, or sodium content to make foods more addictive, many are marking their products gluten-free. Just because something is gluten-free doesn't mean that it is safe. Many gluten-free options contain far too many carbohydrates. We need roughly 60 to 80 grams of carbohydrates a day. Be careful about getting 40 grams from one gluten-free muffin or 20 from a handful of gluten-free crackers.

- Truly organic foods will be more expensive, but also much more nutritious. According to Professor Carlo Leifert of the Tesco Center for Organic Agriculture, organic fruits and vegetables have up to 40 percent more antioxidants than non-organically grown produce, while organic milk contains up to 60 percent more antioxidants and healthy fatty acids than conventional milk.[2] In other words, you are getting about twice the nutrition for only a little bit more money. Pound for pound, that makes organics worth it.

- It's not only that these foods are more nutritious, but they are also less toxic. Truly organic foods have had no artificial fertilizers used on the soil, no pesticides added, and no hormones, antibiotics, or other chemicals or drugs added to enhance growth or bolster weak systems. Healthy plants and animals will have systems strong enough to resist disease and insects on their own.

- Humane treatment of animals is also a priority for those seeking to be truly organic. Free-range is better than cage-free, and wild-caught fish is much preferred over farm-raised fish.

- Be as informed as possible about where your meats, dairy, and eggs are coming from and what those animals were fed. Don't eat meats from animals that eat foods you wouldn't eat. This means choosing grass-fed or green-fed beef over grain-fed. Also, find out what antibiotics, steroids, or other drugs or chemicals were given to the animals while they were being raised.

While this list probably seems a little overwhelming at first, remember, we are running a marathon here, not a sprint. All of this doesn't have to be done in a day—or even a week—especially if you have children taking issue with suddenly seeing asparagus instead of chicken nuggets on their plates. I have two simple rules for transitioning toward healthier meals:

1. First, simply add more healthy foods and drinks rather than taking anything away.

2. Second, replace rather than just eliminate. Herbal teas or water for sodas, organic (or raw) milk for reduced-fat milks, organic fruits for pre-packaged snacks.

DID YOU KNOW?

Statistically we spend a *smaller percentage* of our net income on groceries than ever before. Just in the last 30 years, American spending on groceries has gone down from more than 12 percent to less than 9 percent according to the Bureau of Labor and Statistics.

Change Your Food; Change Your Life!

Epigenetics is the study of how the potentiality or the expression of genes in the human body can be changed. It is the study of the "soup" surrounding our genes. This "soup" decides which chemicals get switched on and which chemicals get switched off. And we can change the messages sent from our brains to our cells via this powerful, genetic soup. Did you get that? We are not controlled by fate or our inherited tendencies! We have the power to change our lives by changing our gene expression and the potential of future gene function! This relatively new scientific field of epigenetics is integrally tied to human choice. We as humans have been given the great gift of being able to choose whether we will eat for health or eat for merely pleasure. We can choose whether to be grateful or bitter. We can choose whether to allow the winds of life to beat us down, or whether to let them lift us up so we can soar. With this gift comes awesome responsibility.

One of the simplest ways that we can change our genetic potential is through what we eat. When we are consistently mindful about getting the right nutrients into our bodies, then we will begin to see amazing benefits in every area of our lives. How can I make this bold statement? Because I have seen those who have changed their "gut biomes." This in turn led to better mental and physical health. With more stamina and energy, those persons began to think more clearly, make better life choices, and take advantage of opportunities they would have previously avoided or not even recognized. Those opportunities then propelled them financially and socially to places they never thought they would be. Changing your eating will change your life!

What does this look like on a daily basis? At first it will look like baby steps. When you meet someone for lunch, you may decide to go somewhere where you can get a salad instead of a heavy, carb-laden sandwich or pasta entrée. Later in your journey it may look like having a first meal of eggs, avocado, mushrooms, tomatoes, and spinach later in the morning. It will look like having the equivalent of three platefuls of vegetables each and every day, and eating full-fat cream and butter instead of a fake butter substitute. For now I want you to get that *you* are in charge of your health, and your choices today affect your genetic expression tomorrow!

#2) HYDRATE

Survivalists abide by the "rule of threes": other than in rare cases, humans can survive for three minutes without air, three hours in freezing temperatures, three days without water, and three weeks without food. The fact that water is the third most vital element on this list, behind air and warmth, is no small thing. We as humans are dependent on a clean, reliable supply of water, and we need it several times a day.

Water benefits the entire body. It irrigates cells so that they can efficiently process all that you consume, keeps the engine of digestion running smoothly, and lowers body temperature in stifling heat. It increases your metabolism allowing it to burn more calories, and it hydrates the cardiovascular system. Water also helps the liver and kidneys flush out wastes at the end of the digestive process.[3] Our lungs are 90 percent water, our brains are 70 percent water, our blood is more than 80 percent water, and our entire bodies are roughly 65 percent water. No wonder it is so vital to human health!

How much water is enough? Although you can *survive* on less, in order to *thrive*, you should be drinking half your body weight (pounds) in ounces of pure, filtered water each day. So if you weigh 150 pounds, you should be drinking 75 ounces of water. There are eight ounces in a cup, so that means consuming roughly nine and a half cups per day.

JUICING VS. BLENDING

Juicing is a fast way to get nutrients into your system. Juicers remove the fiber—which we don't digest anyway—from the fruits and vegetables; leaving all of the essential nutrients—macro- and micronutrients—of whatever you fed through the juicer. Vegetable juices are great for healing, nourishing, and rejuvenating your body at a cellular level. They give you all of the benefits of the whole vegetables and fruits without the stress of passing the fiber through your digestive system. The nutrients are absorbed more quickly than they would be if you either put the same produce into a smoothie or soup, or ate it as part of a meal. The downside of this is that because they are more quickly absorbed, you are also likely to get hungry again in a shorter amount of time. Most people who do juice fasts tend to "eat" more often, so they don't want to be far from their juicers.

Juicing should also be restricted to mostly vegetables with some fruit—usually apple, mixed in for contrast and to help the juicing process. If you juice mostly fruit, you are throwing a bunch of sugar into your system without the benefit of the fruit's fiber to slow the absorption. Believe it or not, the sugar in fruit juice and sugar in a soda pop affect your body in almost exactly the same way.

An added benefit of some juicers is that you can collect the pulp from what is juiced, dry it, and use it in gluten-free baking mixed with some other gluten-free flour.

Blending fruits, vegetables, nuts, etc. into smoothies or soups means you are still getting the whole food—nutrients and fiber—plus additional liquid. The fiber then slows the digestive process, releasing the nutrients into your system little by little over a longer time. Chances are you will then find a smoothie filling for three to four hours and a juice for one or two, though of course, that will vary depending on your digestion and what you are putting into your juicer or blender.

Smoothies are also better for fruits, though I would still suggest using mostly fruits that have a low glycemic index (GI) like blueberries, strawberries, and blackberries. Our systems just don't need that much sugar, especially if one of your goals is to burn fat.

In this light, smoothies are a better option for your first meal of the day because they will keep you satisfied longer, and you can get protein into them easily by adding nuts, seeds, or a good quality whey protein powder. Juices are better if you feel like you just can't get in all the vegetable servings you should have in a day because it is just too much to eat. Juices can also be a great late afternoon or evening snack to give you a boost when you are only an hour or two from your next (or last) meal, or when you are feeling tired and want quick energy without drinking caffeine. Juicing is also always a great part of any detox plan.

Avoid mixing starchy vegetables (carrots, zucchini, broccoli, etc.) with fruits as they will often ferment in your stomach and give you gas. Leafy greens, however, can be combined with just about anything.

Smoothies, juices, soups, etc. made with either juicers or blenders should be eaten within 15 minutes of being made, if possible, to get their maximum nutritional benefits.

Not all waters are equal. Numerous studies have shown that tap water is a major source of toxic chemicals and adds toxic stress to your liver and kidneys. Many bottled waters have pictures of pristine mountains and clear streams on them, promising to be from natural springs or have special qualities. However, at least a third of them are simply filtered tap water! Few, in fact, are worth the plastic containers they are delivered in. Yet bottled water is still a $4 billion-a-year industry that charges us roughly 1,900 percent more than if we simply got water from our own taps. If our nation were to spend an equal amount of money that is spent on producing, consuming, and then handling the waste from bottled water, we could easily have cleaner water systems for people the world over. The practical solution is to get a water filter for the home and office and always drink your water from that in a reusable, BPA-free cup or bottle.[4]

EVOLUTION VS. REVOLUTION

Step 1: Drinking little to no pure water

Step 2: Replacing sodas and coffee with water and caffeine-free herbal teas each day

Step 3: Always have a glass of filtered water near you during the day and drink from it every time you think of it

Step 4: Drinking half your body weight in ounces of pure, filtered water

And water is not just for drinking. Clean water is also important for bathing and showering every day. Water works as a natural stimulus increasing energy and resistance to disease. Because we are warm-blooded, we react to changes in temperature, and these reactions activate all the vital body systems to equalize and stabilize body functions. Cool or cold water stimulates our bodies and increases the use of oxygen in our cells. Bathing in warm or hot water stimulates blood vessels and improves circulation. That, in turn, improves the transportation of oxygen to the cells and brain and speeds up the elimination of toxins. *Hydrotherapy*, as many call it—therapy through water—can inspire not only a well-balanced body, but also a healthy, alert mind.[5]

#3) SUPPLEMENT WISELY

While the majority of nutrition should come from our food, good nutritional supplements are incredibly beneficial. Just as we want our diet to be centered on whole, living foods, any supplements that we take should also come from whole, living foods as well.

Myth:

Calories are calories—they are all the same.

Truth:

Food that has been made by man or altered by man has calories that act differently in your body than foods that are natural and that we have been eating for thousands of years.

Supplements are important because they can give us nutrients that aren't readily available in our modern world. Things like sodium, potassium, magnesium, and calcium are electrolytes that carry electrical charges throughout our bodies. They also dissolve completely into water so that they are easily transported to wherever our bodies need them the most. Our cells communicate with our brains using these electrically-charged particles. Because of the contamination of our fish supply with mercury, it is wise to include a good quality omega-3 supplement every day. Most Americans are deficient in vitamin D_3 because of the amount of time we spend indoors, our dietary choices, and our overuse of sunscreens. Because vitamin D is really a hormone, not a vitamin, it is important to make sure your levels are adequate. This will most likely require supplementation. Optimal dosage is 4,000 IUs for adults, and 3,000 IUs for kids 3-8.

Our bodies need to maintain a delicate balance between sodium and potassium for communication between the brain and the cells to be clear and effective. To put it in simplest terms, sodium pumps water into our cells while potassium pumps waste products out. Too much sodium and we tend toward fluid retention, puffiness, and high blood pressure. Because of the high level of sodium we typically get in our normal diets, the issue is usually getting enough potassium to keep sodium in balance. To maintain this balance, when we don't get enough potassium in what we eat, our kidneys will work overtime trying to find enough potassium to send our cells what they need. A similar balance is needed for calcium and magnesium. In the standard American diet we tend to get more than enough calcium and not enough magnesium. To get more magnesium, we need to eat a diet richer in leafy, green vegetables and nuts.

DID YOU KNOW?

Kale has the most nutrition per calorie of any plant on earth.

We don't have enough space here to go into all of the different needs our bodies have for supplements, and those needs are unique to each individual. However, in the world of industrialized nutrition, widespread antibiotic use, and indoor workplaces, it is fairly safe to say that most North Americans can benefit from starting with these three supplements: omega-3, vitamin D_3, and probiotics (healthy, helpful bacteria).

KEEP IT SIMPLE, KEEP IT FUN

One of the great things coming out of the real food movement is not just the reclaiming of health, but also the reclaiming of our kitchens and the joy of cooking. Food has always been a social connector. From Thanksgiving dinner to soccer team potlucks, food has always connected us. It is the constant tradition in a world of change. Finding ways to cook fresh vegetables adding grass-fed, free-range meats and wild-caught fish and replacing breads and grains with more healthful options doesn't need to change that connection. In fact, it will keep us around longer to enjoy those connections with the ones we love!

To say it won't be different, however, would be disingenuous. These new habits will require changing our way of thinking as well as the time needed for planning. Learning to time our evenings better will be essential. Taking time to cook sweet potatoes in the oven, taking the meat out of the freezer to thaw in the morning, preparing dishes before we cook them, leaving things overnight to soak or marinate, using the slow cooker more often—all of this takes more time. This will be different than walking into the kitchen 10 or 15 minutes before mealtime, opening something prepackaged, and just following the directions on the box. The greatest assets you have are your health and your time. They go hand in hand. Investing them synergistically will give you great fulfillment and more joy in life.

Eating more healthfully is going to take more planning and creativity, but there is no reason for it to become burdensome. And there is no reason it has to be left all to mom either. While being around the dinner table and having a family meal is a powerful bonding time, cooking together can be just as powerful. Involving kids in this process helps them to appreciate what they are eating, and reduces complaining once it is served. It also educates them about healthy food choices, teaches them about cooking, and builds their sense of competency. Having your kids shop with you and teaching them to read labels can take this even further.

As with any new process, this might not be easy at first; but like most activities we share with our children, in the end it will create treasured memories to be passed on for generations. Most modern parents share too little of their regular household "chores" with their kids, and miss the benefits of bonding time, the opportunity to teach responsibility, and the creation of a sense of family.

EVOLUTION VS. REVOLUTION

Step 1:   Regular sodas

Step 2:   Sports drinks with electrolytes

Step 3:   Juicer juices that are mostly vegetables

Step 4:   Most of our hydration comes from pure, filtered water

Another component of the real food movement that creates opportunities for connection is "farm-to-table," which epitomizes the desire to not only know where our food is coming from, but to take part in producing it. This farm-to-table tradition involves taking our families to cooperative farms to contribute time or share the experience of creating, caring for, and harvesting from our own backyard gardens. You may not have time for all these different activities, but you can pick and choose the ones that will work for you and that you can enjoy with your family. Simply going to a "pick your own" apple farm as a family is a delightful experience that children love and appreciate. Keeping them alongside you to help make homemade applesauce when you get home is something they will never forget.

Reconnecting with the food we eat is important, not just for community and health, but for wholeness. There is a morality of stewardship that comes from reconnecting with the food we eat and the ground in which it is grown or upon which it is raised. Like so many things, attitude is important. We have the freedom of choice to make anything fun or tedious, and there are powerful benefits to learning how to have fun and choose to enjoy every task we undertake. We always have a choice, and choosing to live in joy as much as possible not only makes life more fun, but has powerful health benefits as well.

NOTES

1. "Obesity and Overweight," *World Health Organization* fact sheet, (updated: August 2014), http://www.who.int/mediacentre/factsheets/fs311http://www.who.int/mediacentre/factsheets/fs311/en//en/ (accessed: September 11, 2014).

2. "Beyond Organic Coach Program," Beyond Organic handout, 11.

3. Rubin, *The Maker's Diet Revolution,* 59.

4. "The 6 Worst Brands of Bottled Water You Can Buy," Mercola .com (January 21, 2011), http://articles.mercola.com/sites/articles/archive/2011/01/21/best-and-worst-bottled-water-brands.aspx (accessed September 25, 2014).

5. Gursche, Siegfried, *Encyclopedia of Natural Healing* (Richmond, BC, Canada: Alive Publishing Group, Inc., 1997), 347.

Step Eight

Gratitude

People who laugh actually live longer
than those who don't laugh. Few
persons realize that health actually varies
according to the amount of laughter.
—JAMES J. WALSH

Be joyful because it is humanly possible.
—WENDELL BERRY

Recently I made a friend who for almost a decade lived in Greece, the land of the Mediterranean diet based on fresh vegetables, olive oil, and goat cheese, with watermelon and cantaloupe for dessert. He told me about how the Modern Greek language is still littered with phrases from early Christianity. One of his favorites is a traditional greeting pronounced *hyair-e-tay*. It means "rejoice."

As he explains it, in the Greek language the words for joy and grace are very similar and have similar roots. The word *grace* has the sense of "unmerited favor," but also implies having more than enough of whatever—energy, ability, time, resources, patience— enough for oneself *and* enough to spare for others. It means that no matter what is happening, there is a margin between where you are at the moment and being maxed out. In other words, you always have a little extra just in case you need it. Choosing to live by joy is a key to having that kind of grace. It is very closely related to having rest and recovery built into your life so that you are not always operating at 110 percent. It is a lifestyle change that, although difficult to master, will actually give you more energy and vitality in the long run.

Choosing to have the right attitude and having this kind of "margin" in your life oils the gears of relationships, human inter- actions, and ultimately society at large. Believe it or not, it also oils internal functions and helps you adapt to and recover from the stresses in your life. Those who have grace have room to be both generous and grateful, no matter what is happening around them. They choose to live by what is important rather than getting lost in what is urgent or dramatic. It is an attitude that makes life bet- ter for everyone.

So, when Greek villagers greet each other saying, "Rejoice!" it isn't a religious duty. They are actually reminding one another of the importance of being joyful—and of this creation and recogni- tion of grace in their lives. They are reminding one another that the best things in life bring joy and that ultimately, *joy is a choice.* Not a bad thing to remind ourselves of everyday, don't you think? Wouldn't you rather be around people who create an environment of joy, grace, and hope rather than those who constantly fill the atmosphere with conflict, criticism, and despair?

JOY IS A CHOICE

A great deal of modern stress comes from our mental thoughts and emotional feelings. Feelings are ruled by beliefs and thoughts, so when we get our thoughts and beliefs grounded in truth, our emotions will be more steady and positive. How hopeful and confident we are in our own power to make a difference in the world has a tremendous bearing on the body's stress response. Joy is a choice and a habit of being. The cultivation of gratitude and joy is the way home. It is the way to create rest and peace in your life no matter how chaotic the circumstances that surround you. Joy is the most terrifying and difficult emotion that we experience, because when we allow ourselves to feel joy, we immediately tap into a primal fear that someone or something is bound to take that joy away from us. The great thing about building our joy on the eternal things that don't fade is that no one can take that away from us. If our joy is not centered on our circumstances, then any change in our circumstances won't alter our joy. It will be an artesian well springing up within us that bubbles forth with a steady stream, clear and pure.

The four areas that work together to determine our overall outlook on life are:

- What we think

- What we feel

- What we say

- What we do

What We Think

What we allow ourselves to think about directly affects the limbic system. This is the region of our brains that controls emotions, memories, heart rate, blood pressure, and attention span. How we think about life affects how positive and happy we are, regardless of our circumstances, and that in turn facilitates or hinders limbic function. We may not be able to control our circumstances, but we can certainly control our attitudes and responses to them.

Are you a glass half-full or a glass half-empty type of person? Do you forgive easily, or do you hang on to grudges until you can get even in some way? Are you a victor or a victim? These are important questions, because these attitudes have a direct effect on how stress will impact every cell in your body. A person with a purpose in life who knows his reason for being here can weather a great many storms without them directly influencing his health. While this doesn't give you permission to burn the candle at both ends, it is important to consider your outlook as a crucial factor directly related to your ability to adapt to and recover from stress—the silent killer.

WAKE-UP CALL

Cynics have more than a two-and-a-half-time greater risk of developing dementia than those who have gratitude.

Cynical distrust is described as believing that most people are self-interested and out for themselves as opposed to looking out for the community and others. Some experts describe cynicism as chronic anger—anger that simmers on the back burner for a lifetime.

What We Feel

Scientists have told us for quite some time that our moods affect our health. However, the underlying cellular mechanisms of how this happens were murky until researchers began looking at gene-expression profiles inside white blood cells. Gene expression is the complex process by which genes direct the production of proteins. These proteins jump-start other processes, which, in the case of white blood cells, control much of the body's immune response.

A recent study on health and happiness found that subjects who focused on finding happiness in their own comfort and pleasure had remarkably unhealthy cellular profiles as well as high levels of inflammation in their systems. They also had lower levels of antibody production. In contrast, those who sought happiness through helping others had lower readings for inflammatory factors in their blood, and they produced more antibodies. In other words, *why* we are happy matters as much as *actually* being happy.

What We Say

How we speak to others often portrays thoughts and attitudes we never realized we had. Are you generally a grateful person, or are you one who fears that others are trying to take advantage of you? Are you polite or surly? Do you take the time needed to be considerate of others, or do you always cut to the chase? Is your "to do list" more important than what other people think or how they feel? There are numerous studies on the importance of having an attitude of gratitude in all things. How you express gratitude and appreciation impacts your health in very direct ways. Grateful people are peaceful people. Peaceful people are joyful people. Joyful people are generally healthy people in mind, body, and spirit. Gratitude is a habit. To become better at it, we must practice it each and every day.

What We Do

Selfish actions are at the root of all kinds of misery. It is important to us on multiple levels to live for a higher purpose than merely our own pleasure. Having a higher calling and acting according to this calling in service to others makes a huge difference to genetic expression. According to an article in *New York Magazine*:

> Our genes may have a more elevated moral sense than our minds do, according to a new study of the genetic effects of happiness. They can, it seems, reward us with healthy gene activity when we're unselfish—and chastise us, at a microscopic level, when we put our own needs and desires first.[1]

To give yourself an idea of how healthy or unhealthy your thoughts, attitudes and actions are, consider the answers to these five questions:

1. How often do you feel depleted and empty physically, mentally, or emotionally?

2. How often do you feel that your life circumstances are spiraling out of control?

3. How much would it take to push you over the edge?

4. Do you find yourself becoming angry over seemingly small things?

5. Do you need a vacation to recuperate from your vacation?

If the answers to these questions alarm you, maybe it's time to do some reevaluating of how you are operating in your life. What are you going to do so that you have the physical, mental, and emotional rest you need to keep stress from taxing you beyond your limits? What adjustments can you make? What recuperation and capacity-building activities can you add to your routine to give yourself an outlet for stress? When will you allow your body to repair and recover from the stress that is killing most Americans today?

GRACE UNDER PRESSURE

We need to learn to run our lives so that we aren't always pushing as hard as we can, running to our limit and beyond. The tendency to do that is exactly the type of lifestyle Richard Swenson prescribes a remedy for in his book, *Margin: Restoring Emotional, Physical, Financial, and Time Reserves to Overloaded Lives*. Swenson uses the word *margin* in a way that is similar to how I have used the word *grace* in this chapter: It's about always believing that you have more than enough, about being able to be gracious because you live in abundance, and about keeping a marked distance between where you are operating and your absolute limits. To have *margin* or *grace* is to have more than enough left over; to be "margin less" is to use up what you have and then extract more from others in order to make up the difference. As he puts it:

> Margin less is being 30 minutes late to the doctor's office because you were 20 minutes late getting out of the bank because you were ten minutes late dropping the kids off at school because your car ran out of gas two blocks from the gas station—and you forgot your wallet....
>
> Margin less is fatigue; margin is energy.
>
> Margin less is red ink; margin is black ink.

Margin less is hurry; margin is calm.

Margin less is anxiety; margin is security.

Margin less is culture; margin is counterculture.

Margin less is the disease of the new millennium; margin is its cure.[2]

We must never forget that we are in charge of our reactions—we always have a choice in how we respond to the circumstances the world throws at us. We can choose to leave a little extra room, or we can choose to live life running along—and often hanging over—the edge. We can choose being joyful or fretting about our circumstances; choose saving or spending; choose real foods over ones that delight our taste buds but have little to no nutritional value. We can choose people over things; choose gratitude over envy; choose pleasantness over irritability; choose exercise over lethargy; choose sleep over one more hour of channel surfing; choose getting ahead little by little over falling behind; and so on and so forth. We can choose to live with something left over all of the time—with margin or grace—or spend everything we have and then borrow more from someone else thinking we will make it up later—which very few of us ever do.

BEING JOYFUL MEANS "YOU NEVER HAVE TO LET THEM SEE YOU SWEAT"

The great thing about this is that everything becomes easier when you live with grace, even though it may be a hard habit to develop at the beginning. It means doing without *now* so that you have plenty *later.* It means setting your limits far away from the edge of a cliff. Many people see limits as constraints, but to the creative, limits are really freedom. It means doing what Dave

Ramsey advises: "Live [now] like no one else, so that you can later live—and give—like no one else." Grace—having margin or extra—is the basis for generosity, for helping others, and for living for something beyond your own comfort and satisfaction. As we have said before, this is the key to *true* happiness.

Let me give you an example. There was once a grade school building along a busy highway, and the playground of the school had one edge that ran right along that thoroughfare. Cars and trucks whizzed by at 60 or 70 miles an hour. As a result, kids played far back away from the highway, using only about half of the playground. Eventually, though, the school district built a guardrail and fence between the highway and the playground. Do you know what happened? Kids began using the entire playground for the first time, feeling it was safe to go right up to the edge of the fence without fear of getting too close to the traffic. The limit of that fence gave them more freedom; not less.

The same happens with money. Have you ever noticed how couples argue less when they have a budget they have agreed upon? If two have agreed together that they will allocate so much for personal spending and one of them goes out and buys something the other thinks is ridiculous, will they argue over it like they did before? Probably not. Why? Because they know they will still have money for the other things in their life because they have set limits to protect their overall needs. They have also set boundaries on what is their own discretionary spending and what is their spouse's.

Choosing to have a grateful and joyful attitude will have a similar effect. It gives us margin between where we normally operate and what will drive us over the edge. It means setting boundaries on what we will allow to frazzle us and how we will react when we are challenged. Now I know you may be thinking, "Oh, if it were only that easy!" I know what you mean. It's going to take some time to step back, see what is happening, and decide ahead of time that you are going to find a new routine for the common cues that have driven you over the edge in the past. It is going to force you to find ways of responding that will give you time to collect yourself and be positive, even in the face of negativity or crisis. It's not easy, but it is simple; and when you do it, you will soon find people respecting you for it.

As an example, I once knew a middle-aged woman, with seven grown children, who had been overweight for most of her adult life. There were many reasons for her lack of health, not the least of which was that she drank two or three cans of Pepsi each and every day. Over the course of her lifetime, she had ingested hundreds of thousands of teaspoons of sugar just from these drinks. They became such an idol in her life that if anyone even touched her cans on the porch, she would say, "Who's been in my drinks?" It became a family joke.

As she neared 60 she suffered from digestive issues, crippling arthritis, joint pain, fatigue, and high blood sugar. Then she decided to get serious. In her 60s she underwent gastric bypass surgery and lost 100 pounds. Her blood sugar returned to normal, her arthritis began to heal, and she began to be able to walk up and down their long and winding driveway out in rural Minnesota. Did the surgery do this? Not really. She got counseling at the same time and was told that she needed to address her reactions to the stressors in her life. Finances, relationships, anger management, disappointments—all these were triggers that caused pain. She buried and numbed the pain with sugar. Now she had to do things differently, or she would surely die. So she did. And after a couple of years, no one remembered the "fat" lady or the lady addicted to the sugary drinks. What they saw was a woman under control. A woman who laughed a lot and could walk pretty darn fast for her age! Everyone began to respect her for who she had become. Not so much because of the weight loss, but they respected her because she could deal with her emotions in a mature, adult manner—not hiding behind an aluminum can.

In this way, living with margin in every area of your life will improve your relationships, your sense of purpose, your sense of fulfillment, and your overall health. A pretty good bargain really. It means you will handle difficulties and the storms of life with maturity—truly exhibiting grace under pressure.

THERE'S A BETTER WAY

The following is a list of behaviors that characterize chronically unhappy people.

Check in with yourself to see if any of these feel familiar.

1. Your default belief is that life is hard.

2. You believe that most people can't be trusted.

3. You spend more time focusing on what's wrong in your life than what's right.

4. You compare yourself to others and harbor jealousy or envy.

5. You seek to control.

6. You think about your future with worry and fear.

7. You fill your conversations with gossip and complaining.

Many people feel like they have no hope, and you may be one of them. You may have read this chapter and figured I am just some kind of Pollyanna—being unrealistically positive. You know better though. Why? Think back to the stories I have already shared in this book. Are your problems any bigger than the ones they faced? Probably not—different, yes, but not bigger.

Science has shown us that the human brain is by design neuroplastic—it is able to adapt and respond to new ways of doing things. When you understand how neural pathways are created in the brain, you will truly comprehend how to let go of bad habits like overeating or worry, ingratitude or cynicism, burning the candle at both ends, or habitually neglecting your own self-care. Neural pathways are like superhighways of nerve cells that transmit messages. You travel over the superhighway many times, and the pathway becomes more and more solid. You may go to a specific food or cigarettes for comfort over and over, and that forms a brain pathway. The hopeful fact is that the brain is always changing, and you can forge new pathways and create new habits. Because of this marvelous quality of neuroplasticity (the brain's ever-changing potential) anything is possible. Did you hear that? Anything. Is. Possible.

That is why I want you to know that you are not without hope. The power to get healthier and live the life your heart desires is possible. How do I know? Because I have seen so many do it. I have seen people make new choices and through them create the life they have always wanted. If you are not there yet, then it is because you need to learn more, you need to develop new strengths or skills, or you need to find someone who will team up with you and help you stay on track. Basically you need to form some new superhighways in that marvelous brain of yours. Once again, that is exactly what Unhealthy Anonymous is all about—moving forward together to do what we were put on the earth to do.

NOTES

1. Gretchen Reynolds, "Looking to Genes for the Secret to Happiness," NYTimes.com, (this article originally appeared in the *New York Times Magazine*, August 25, 2013), http://well.blogs .nytimes.com/2013/08/23/what-our-genes-reveal-about-true -happiness/ (accessed September 28, 2014).

2. Richard A. Swenson, *Margin: Restoring Emotional, Physical, Financial, and Time Reserves to Overloaded Lives* (Colorado Springs, CO: Navpress, 2004), 13.

Step Nine

Movement

Lack of activity destroys the good
condition of every human being, while
movement and methodical physical
exercise save it and preserve it.
—PLATO

Jann walked into her first Unhealthy Anonymous meeting with the help of a cane. Though she was only in her 60s, she felt as if she were 120. Her arthritis hurt so much she could barely accomplish a fraction of what she once handled with ease. In fact, she was forced to retire from her job because the continual standing—six to eight hours a day for two or three days at a time—was just too much. She moved slowly and methodically into the room, looking carefully for a chair at the end of one of the rows.

Though she wasn't sure of what to expect, soon after the first speaker was introduced, she sat in amazement at what she was hearing. Why hadn't she heard anything like this about "real food" before? There was so much to learn! Unknowingly she had been buying foods steeped in antibiotics, growth hormones, and an assortment of harmful chemicals. What had she been doing to herself and her family all of these years?

As she listened, she learned about the benefits of coconut oil, grass-fed beef, organic produce, and about the power of healthy foods to reduce inflammation and give our systems the energy they need to make us healthy and strong. One of her favorite presentations, called "Shopping with the Doc," gave her helpful tips that virtually changed her buying and eating habits overnight.

When she got home, she immediately implemented what she'd learned that night. She began faithfully working her way through the phases of the program. As she got to phase three, the pounds began to fall off. First 10…then 20…30…40…50…and so on. She fell in love with the recipes provided at the workshop, and she began to create her own. Over time her body improved dramatically, and since then she has had no desire to go back to the way she had been feeding herself and her family before.

She admits that it was hard to resist cooking her family's former favorite meals, especially at holiday gatherings, so she found clever ways to convert those old favorites to healthy dishes. Sometimes she still bakes and decorates traditional birthday cakes for her grandkids' birthday parties. The difference is she's never tempted to lick the spoon after she has frosted the cake or sneak a secret slice at one of the parties. There is simply no way she wants to go back to feeling the way she did. After all, if she really wanted a treat, she could always make something healthy like raw cacao almond butter cups or avocado chocolate mousse—yum!

EVOLUTION VS. REVOLUTION

Step 1: Dessert every night or sweets between meals
Step 2: Substitute fruit for dessert and snacks
Step 3: Stop eating by 7:00 every night; desserts only on the weekends
Step 4: Healthy desserts on special occasions only

While her weight loss currently isn't as dramatic as it was in the beginning, Jann's arthritis is no longer an issue, and she no longer walks with a cane. She might, however, use a walking stick when she goes for a hike in the mountains to capture a scene for an upcoming watercolor. Taking up painting was something she hadn't thought possible with the way her hands had hurt before, but now it is one of her favorite activities. Her health has improved so much that her former employer offered her the old job back. Physically, she could have easily returned, but instead her answer was, "Absolutely not...I'm having too much fun doing what I do now!" By changing her eating, she changed her life! Losing her job had at one time seemed like a great loss, but with renewed health and energy, Jann was able to clearly see and take advantage of new and better opportunities.

THE NEED FOR SPINAL MOVEMENT

Because the brain and the spine are the central command for the rest of the body, it is very important that their communication channels be clear and unimpeded. Likewise when these two "talk" to the cells, they need paths of clear communication. When you were a child playing hide-and-go-seek after dark, did you ever hide so well that you couldn't hear the "All ye all ye in come free?"

You stayed there wondering in the dark whether it were truly safe to run to "home base." Spinal adjustments are what allow all your cells to hear the call that they indeed may return to a place of rest and homeostasis.

How does this happen? Proprioception is a sensory receptor network found chiefly in muscles, tendons, joints, and the inner ear that detects the motion or position of the body by responding to stimuli arising with the organism. The stimulus in this case would be the specific spinal adjustment. The proprioceptive input from restoring spinal alignment and the proper range of motion leads to sensory input into the cerebellar-brainstem-cortical loops that coordinate movement, muscle tone, and posture as well as learning, emotions, and basic bodily functions.

Many fields of study including neuroscience, neurophysiology, endocrinology, psychoneuroimmunology, and education support the fact that proprioception is an essential nutrient for proper brain and nervous system function. In other words, the movement associated with specific spinal alignment and mobility is necessary for your brain and nerves to return to a place of rest and balance. Nobel Prize recipient Dr. Roger Sperry says that the spine is the motor that drives the brain. According to his research "90% of the stimulation and nutrition to the brain is generated by the movement of the spine."

THE NEED FOR REGULAR, SPECIFIC EXERCISE

Until recently I figured all exercise was pretty much the same. I mean what's the difference between running, walking, playing tennis or racquetball, riding your bike, jumping on a rebounder, or getting on the treadmill? Sure, some are more intense than others, but as long as you are moving, they all benefit the body similarly, don't they? The truth is, however, they don't. Yes, all of them benefit you, but one is better than all the rest.

As it turns out, the most effective way to burn fat and maintain a healthy body weight is an exercise regimen called "burst training" or high intensity interval training (HIIT for short). Not only is it the most effective exercise, but it won't cut into your busy schedule as much as other programs will. Why? Because it takes only 15 minutes to do, five or six times a week.

HIIT is based on alternating back and forth between periods of working at or near maximum effort with rest. So, instead of taking a 30-minute walk, you would do intervals alternating between a minute of running (high intensity) and a minute of walking (rest and recovery) for a total of ten minutes. The workout takes a third the time, but makes a greater impact on your health. Or you could do the same activity in a pool, which is easier on your joints.

Exercise is great for a number of reasons. While we know it is good for burning calories and developing muscles, did you know it also reduces chronic pain? According to a study by Harvard researchers, women suffering from fibromyalgia improved their strength and endurance while reducing their pain through 20 weeks of regular exercise.

Exercise also detoxifies the body. As we move and exert our muscles, we increase *peristalsis*—the "squeezing" movements that work with our endocrine systems to remove waste from our bodies. When we exercise, we sweat out toxins through our skin and strengthen our arteries and veins. Muscles also hold less fluid than fat cells, so by decreasing fat and increasing muscle mass we clear out excess "water weight."

Short, intense exercise has repeatedly been shown to reduce levels of cortisol fairly quickly. This in turn keeps blood pressure from spiking which is what normally happens when cortisol is released. Breathing through your nose as much as you can rather than breathing through your mouth also helps keep blood pressure lower.

Exercise positively affects insomnia and depression. A Northwestern University study followed a group of sedentary adults for 16 weeks who had been diagnosed with depression and insomnia. Each day the participants spent some time on treadmills, stationary bikes, and/or elliptical machines. At the end of the study all of the participants showed dramatic improvement in their ability to sleep and in their self-reported outlooks on life.

Exercise has some other rather surprising side benefits as well. It stimulates the production of human growth hormone (HGH), testosterone (for both men and women), and cortisol (the stress hormone). Both HGH and testosterone help build lean muscle, burn fat, increase bone density, support joint function, and increase energy levels. Proper levels of testosterone help with memory, sex drive, and brain function. Activating cortisol through exercise makes us more alert and focused throughout the day. The stress hormone cortisol can be harmful if we get too much of it for too long—it will decrease muscle tissue, increase belly fat, and suppress immune function. This is why we like short duration, high effort exercise. More traditional exercise programs consisting of longer workouts with lower intensity activities decrease HGH and testosterone and increase cortisol levels over time; hormones activated through HIIT exercise have the opposite effect. This is why workouts of shorter duration and higher intensities have recently become much more popular—because they are actually more beneficial!

DEVELOP THE HABIT FIRST, MAKE IT A WORKOUT SECOND

For exercise to accomplish all of this, it has to become a regular habit. Even finding the short amount of time it takes to do a workout like this can be a challenge for most of us—especially if we really don't feel like doing it in the first place! Most people don't get incredibly excited at the thought of working out unless they do it as part of a team or sport.

So, it needs to become such a part of your life—such a matter of habit that you don't really think about it. As we learned earlier, every habit starts with a *cue* that brings on a *routine* from which we get a *reward*. Here are a few suggestions for putting "habit theory" to work for you so that exercise becomes a regular part of your weekly routine:

Make your exercise time right after you get out of bed.

This saves times because you don't have to go to the gym, change clothes, and then shower again before you go back to work or go home for the evening. Another benefit is you might still be too sleepy to figure out a good reason not to work out.

One reason to do this is that your body burns more fat on an empty stomach than it does after you have just eaten. Working out in the morning will help raise your metabolism for the entire day and help you burn more fat over time.

(Note: Some people may feel dizzy or nauseated when they exercise without food in their systems. You have to judge this for yourself. Maybe a smoothie or a light snack before you work out? Find what works for you and make it part of your routine.)

As a cue, lay out your workout gear somewhere you will see it first thing when you wake up. Make it as obvious as you need to—put them right by your toothbrush if you have to!

When you see the cue, think of the reward not the routine.

One of the best ways to overcome the "pain" of working out is to fast forward in your mind to how you will feel after you have worked out. Focus on how much better you will feel after the workout, how much more energy you will have, and how nice the warm water from the shower will feel on your muscles while you are getting ready, and all the way through your workout.

Most goal-setting classes tell you to begin with the end in mind. That is great for the short term as well as for the long term.

Use dynamic stretching exercises to warm up.

You will note a lot of online workouts begin with dynamic stretching for the first part of the workout rather than the traditional static (stretch the muscle and hold it for 20-30 seconds) stretching. This is because most trainers have learned that dynamic stretching is best for getting ready for action, while static stretching is better for cooling down.

Because of this, if you are going to run, for example, start by working through a series of dynamic stretches as you walk. This would mean a slow jog with arm rotations, walking knee hugs, or similar stretches. A quick online search will give you enough of these to develop your own routine.

At first, remember that the routine is more important than the workout itself.

A lot of people work out too hard at the beginning, and then by the third day they are so sore they don't even want to get out of bed, let alone go work out. Instead of going as hard as you can, give yourself a couple of weeks to work into the habit. Let yourself rest when you feel like it, and then jump back in again as soon as you're ready. (There are many different websites with beginner workouts available like DailyBurn.com, FitnessBlender.com, and many more. Many are free or reasonably priced.)

If you want to run, follow running coach Jeff Galloway's "run walk run" method.[1] Start out by running for 30 seconds and then walk for 60 seconds at a vigorous pace. Then run again for 30 seconds and then walk again for 60 seconds. Keep this up until you have completed your course or the time you have allotted to run.

Then, for a couple of days, reduce the amount of time you walk between until you are running for 30 seconds and then walking for 30 seconds. Once you have conquered that, increase your interval lengths to one minute running and one minute vigorously walking. Then increase your time running in comparison to your time walking—two minutes running to one walking; then a few days later, three minutes running to one walking. Three minutes of dynamic stretching, three three-to-one intervals, and then three minutes of cool down will give you a 15-minute workout.

Obviously you could try this with swimming, water walking, bike riding, or other activities as well. The general principle is to start easy and work your way up as working out becomes a regular habit for you.

If you haven't walked in years, and if running seems like a highly unattainable goal, don't be discouraged! You can use these techniques just as effectively to begin a walking routine that will benefit you every bit as much as running. You can walk/rest in intervals, increasing the amount of walking time and decreasing the amount of resting time as you feel comfortable. While you are "resting," stretch your arms to the sky, bend over and feel a stretch in the backs of your legs, rotate your torso while leaving your feet planted and your hips stationary. This process may be "two steps forward and one step back," but you will be moving! And you will be moving in the right direction.

EVOLUTION VS. REVOLUTION

Step 1: Little physical activity

Step 2: Walking for a few minutes every day

Step 3: Power walk/run for 12 minutes

Step 4: Add weights for a high intensity interval workout!

Don't start with weight-loss goals, because when you reach your ideal weight, what are you going to do, quit? Instead, align your goals with working into a routine as mentioned above, and then set goals about how many times a week you are going to work out as well as how many times a month. If you want to work up to running a race, find a schedule that would be used by someone training for that race and follow it. (These can easily be found online.)

Remember the guidelines for SMART goals:

- **S**—make it *Specific*;

- **M**—make it *Measurable*;

- **A**—make it *Attainable*;

- **R**—create *Reasonable* steps from where you are now to where you want to be; and

- **T**—give it a *Time frame*.

Setting goals using this formula will help motivate you to stick to your workouts.

Recovery time is as important as exercise time.

While exercise is good for you, time to recover and for your body to strengthen itself is just as important—in fact, it may be more important. Remember the optimum time for working out is less than 30 minutes of high intensity interval training (HIIT). Then you should allow roughly 24 hours for your body to recover.

Listen to your body. Warm up and cool down properly. This will help you prevent injuries and help keep you from being sore.

Once you have mastered these basics, it may be time for you to find a workout buddy or group that will help you continue on your path. Remember the power of *connecting* we discussed in step two. It is far easier to be motivated and faithful if you embrace fitness with a friend or accountability partner than if you try to do it alone.

I DARE YOU TO MOVE

American culture today is far more acquainted with the couch potato and armchair quarterback than it is with the octogenarian playing racquet sports or the 70-year-old triathlete. We have come to accept that as we get older, it's time to slow down—but why do we need to do that when it isn't until we get older that we have time to do more? You see, the body is heavily influenced by a law called "move it or lose it." Think of what happens when someone has a cast on his arm. After six weeks of immobility the arm looks like a toothpick. The muscles have shrunk, the elbow joint can't go through full range of motion, and the entire arm is weak. This happens with our population more than ever before because we as a nation sit so very much. We drive to work, we sit at a desk all day, and we check emails and social media at night in between watching our favorite series on television. We move less than ever, and we are shriveling up as a result.

Now I'm not saying you have to go to the extreme of running marathons just because you are getting ready to retire, but I am saying that if you eat and move right, just like Jann, there is no reason your golden years have to be housebound! You deserve to be fit and ready to go on all the adventures you didn't have enough time for when you were younger.

> **"Hey Doc, I'm too busy to get to the gym except on the weekends! How do I stay fit?"**
>
> It is relatively simple to add functional movements to your everyday routine—even if you are busy or don't want to spend money on a gym membership.
>
> Some movements you should be doing every day are: *bending* (stretch palms down to the floor if you have to pick up something you have dropped), *single leg lunges* (walk and take the stairs), *pushing* (lean body weight against your office wall and rip off ten pushups), *rotating your core* (stand while talking on the phone and "do the twist!"), and *pulling* (mow, rake, and sweep instead of paying to have it done).
>
> This will help your wallet as well as your waistline!

Our bodies aren't really designed to break down as we grow older, or at least not to break down as quickly as they commonly do. In some isolated places in the world, it's not uncommon for many people to live to be over 100 and still be clearheaded and active. Take my grandfather, for instance. He lived to a month shy of his 101st birthday, and lived a healthy, active, and vibrant life. Certainly these older folks may not be keeping up with the teenagers, but neither are they senile or bedridden. Our bodies are designed to rejuvenate themselves. In fact, your body completely replaces itself—every cell one at a time—every three years. This fact highlights the importance of cellular input. We all know the saying, "garbage in, garbage out." This applies to cellular reproduction as well. If cells are "birthed" in a stress mode, they will eventually produce more stressed cells. If, however, through human connection, nutrition, hydration, exercise, rest, good thoughts, clear intentions, calm emotions, gratitude, and generosity we are bathing our cells in positive energy, they will reproduce more of the same healthy cells.

So, if our bodies are constantly working to repair and rejuvenate, why do we age? Again, the culprit is stress. It is our enemy; and as I have said before, if we don't know our enemy, we will never taste victory. We age because of prolonged exposure to external and internal stresses. Certainly we will still get older because stress and toxins are inescapable parts of life, but we don't have to age so quickly. Being in our 60s or 70s—even our 80s or 90s—doesn't mean we have to slow down if we don't want to.

Remember the saying, "If you don't move it, you'll lose it!" If you want to live a long, healthy, and happy life, then I would suggest you get a "running start" at growing older gracefully so that your latter years can be as joyful as your earlier years. Remember, there is no joy in living a longer life if you feel lousy for many of those years. Get healthy, stay healthy, be active, and live fully in all of your days. The earlier you start to do that, the easier it will be to maintain as you get older. So why not start today?

NOTE

1. Jeff Galloway, "Run-Walk," Jeff Galloway Training website, http://www.jeffgalloway.com/training/run-walk/ (accessed September 29, 2014).

Step Ten

Alignment

Movement—specifically spinal
movement—generates 90 percent of
stimulation and nutrition to the brain.
—DR. ROGER SPERRY

Anne learned about our office through a booth we set up at the Knoxville Marathon Pick-up Event. She had participated in the 5K run that day and had some balance issues she wanted us to examine. We set up an appointment with her, and she came into our offices a week or so later.

After that she stayed in touch, frequently attending meetings we had in the area. She attended several of our "Shop with the Doc" presentations and learned something new at each event. She also attended a lecture we gave called "The Great Cholesterol Myth" in which we exposed the mistake we make when we avoid healthy fats because we are concerned about raising our cholesterol. Anne got on one of the food programs we shared at that meeting, and as a result was able to discontinue her use of prescription statin drugs. The increased level of quality nutrition going into her body gave her more stamina, energy, strength, and mental clarity.

As she put it:

> Every event helped shape my new lifestyle and made my life more rewarding. I now have healthier eating habits by following your great recipes and am also benefitting from the use of healthier skin and oral care products per your recommendations. My balance disorder has greatly improved since beginning treatment with you. All of these services are being provided by people whom I now consider to be family. I wish more people could take advantage of your services. Thank you!

ALIGN WITH THE RIGHT HEALTH PARADIGM

As we get into the last three steps of the Unhealthy Anonymous program, I want to address one more dichotomy present in the functional medicine approach vs. the traditional medical approach. Many still don't understand that they truly do have the power to be healthy. Far too many have accepted the idea that disease is buried in their genetic code like some kind of ticking time bomb. They believe their health is ruled almost entirely by genetic predisposition; therefore, they believe there is very little they can do to keep from contracting and dying from the same diseases and conditions that afflicted their parents and grandparents.

Family medical history is real, but it's certainly not the whole story. It's true that we get a combination of our mother and father's

DNA, but even geneticists will tell you that health really has very little to do with your gene code. Instead, it has everything to do with *how that gene code is expressed*. The human genome, as we know it, hasn't changed for thousands of years. Everyone likes to talk about genetic mutations, but that belongs far more in the realm of science fiction than it does in reality. The same genes we have now are nearly identical to the genes our ancestors had thousands of years ago. So it isn't our genes that have changed in the last hundred years and brought on the modern-day plague of chronic diseases we are experiencing. It's something else. What has changed is how those genes express themselves—but why?

Most epigenesists will tell you that genetic expression is based on two factors:

1. Your external environment: the air that you breathe, the toxins in your home or workplace, and the general amount of stress you have to face every day.

2. Your responses to the environment: what you choose to eat, how much exercise you get, if you smoke, drink alcohol, are exposed to an overabundance of environmental toxins, and how you manage your stress and emotions.

So, it's not our genes that are changing and bringing on new lifestyle diseases, it's how the same old genes are influenced by our new environments and behaviors. As these two factors change, our genes express themselves differently.

Let me give you an example: Let's say you have a pond in your neighborhood, and one day you pass by it and notice something odd. As you walk up to the water's edge you smell something horrid. Then you see it. There are a whole bunch of dead animals on the shoreline. Now, would you say, "Oh, those animals had a bad family medical history that finally caught up with them?" Or would you think, "There must be something wrong with the pond?" Environment is a much more powerful heath factor than genetic predisposition. That's why it's not all about your genes; it's about your gene expression.

Let me give you a less hypothetical example, and one I have experienced firsthand. Oak Ridge National Laboratory is near Knoxville and is one of the places where parts for the atomic bomb were manufactured. The facility houses a lot of uranium used in their manufacturing, and at one time asbestos was present in many of its buildings. As a result, several people who worked there ended up getting cancer. One particular friend of mine was a chemist who worked there for nearly 30 years. He had several occurrences of cancer. The final occurrence happened while he was nearing 60. We all know that asbestos is a proven external stressor that contributes to cancer. That's not surprising. What *is* surprising is that I also know a number of individuals who worked at Oak Ridge National Laboratory—in the same buildings, drinking the same water, breathing the same air some of them for 20 or more years but they've never had cancer. How is that possible?

This got me thinking. How is it possible that a marathon runner who eats only organic foods and exercises every day of his life drops dead of a heart attack at 37? Yet George Burns lived to be 100 smoking stogies and drinking beer? I've known many individuals who did everything they were supposed to—they ate right, exercised, had regular checkups—but they seemed to die as fast or faster than everyone else. At the same time I've known individuals who eat junk, never work out, and don't do anything that you're supposed to do, yet they seem to live forever.

THE HIDDEN FOURTH FACTOR

So what's the missing variable? Epigenesists tell us the missing variable is the health of the *internal* environment. When you were conceived, you came from two cells—an egg from your mother and sperm from your father—and those cells came together and begin to replicate and duplicate. After only 18 days of replication, they had already formed the most basic part of your brain. This is amazing! Some estimate that the brain produces 65 trillion chemicals a second. Those chemicals are life and instructions for your body, and they are sent out to every cell in your body down your spinal cord. That makes your spinal cord a lifeline of communication.

However, what if, instead of communicating life to every cell of the body, the brain were instead communicating, "Red alert! Red alert! We're under stress! All systems follow emergency protocols!" Now this is helpful when there is an actual emergency, but what about when life and circumstances are just business as usual but our bodies are still getting messages that we are facing crisis? Recent scientific studies have shown that we inherit more than eye and hair color from our parents. We inherit our gut biomes as well. Not only that, but our pattern of adapting to and recovering from stress is set up *in utero*, and it is affected by our mother's emotional state during pregnancy, her exposure to toxins, the foods she eats, and her hormonal balance. We can change our internal terrains through conscious, consistent effort as adults, but by then our bodies have already spent many years adapting and responding to stress in a particular, but not always productive way.

Scientists estimate that our bodies consist of 37.2 trillion cells.[1] Geneticists tell us our brains and bodies are always communicating at a cellular level. When that communication is clear, cells vibrate at a higher rate, and their DNA code expresses itself correctly. Every cell is always doing its best to thrive—to find good nutrients, expelling what it has used up or doesn't need, replicating itself correctly, and getting properly removed at the end of its life cycle without harming any other cells. However, the whole system breaks down when your cells are getting a constant red alert message that they are under attack.

This emergency message can come as a result of many different factors including childhood trauma, sensitivity or an allergy to a particular food you regularly consume, environmental toxins, or even physical cues that trigger memories of stress or trauma. This happens because your limbic system (sometimes called the "reptile brain") controls heart rate, blood pressure, breathing, memory, stress, and other emotions. Certain sights, sounds, and smells can trigger stress in your limbic region, causing the "all alert" to be sounded throughout your body. This is an autonomic response which means that it is totally out of your control. In fact, this stress response may have been inherited from your parents and grandparents! A study done in 2013 showed that mice who were shocked on their feet in response to a certain smell had offspring that had an inborn aversion to that same smell—even though they had never been shocked themselves! We inherit the stress response, but what we do with it is up to us.

Another often overlooked trigger of the stress response is a lack of mobility in what are called the *synovial* joints. Without getting too technical, these include your shoulders, elbows, knees, and spinal vertebrae and discs. When these joints are healthy and have a full range of motion, they activate what are called *mechanoreceptors* that stimulate the cerebellum to send out signals that all is well. This facilitates our body's ability to adapt to and recover from stress. When that mobility is lost, however, synovial joints activate *nociceptors,* which send messages to the brain that stress is present: "*Sound the red alert!*" This loss of motion—even when we are not facing stressors in the world around us—will tell the body to act as if it is being chased by a tiger! Thus, even though all seems well on the outside, our internal mechanisms are often acting as if the tiger is loose. That is why every orthopedic surgeon requires his patients to go through physical therapy after operations on these synovial joints. They know the importance of restoring joint mobility, because restoring proper range of motion restores homeostasis to the body and turns off the stress alarms. The "all clear" message resonating throughout the body facilitates its ability to rest and recover.

CELLULAR HEALTH

Not too long ago I had a businessman enter my office who was something of a genius. He was a physicist and had roughly 1,000 patents. I started explaining the importance of mobility to him, and he asked, "Can I bring some clarity to you?"

"Of course," I said.

So he told me, "Every cell in your body must vibrate to live. Each cell vibrates based on communication to and from the brain by receiving life from it. When a cell vibrates, it allows the DNA of the gene code to express itself correctly. Geneticists have confirmed this. However, if the brain loses communication at the cellular level, the cell's vibrational energy is diminished or slowed down. When that happens, the expression of the gene code becomes altered and mutation occurs." And what do we usually call abnormal or mutated cells? We call them *cancer.* Once again, we see that cancer—like other chronic lifestyle diseases—is more likely to occur in the presence of internal or external stress.

All along, stress has been the hidden enemy of human health and happiness.

This means mobility is essential for the brain to communicate clearly all the way down to the cellular level in order to keep the whole "closed loop" system from sending and receiving distress signals. While the brain runs the body, the spinal cord is the communication trunk sending life-enhancing transmissions to every cell in the body. When the spinal cord is flexible and exhibits proper tone and mobility, the brain communicates efficiently and effectively with your cells at the speed of light. When this happens, every cell vibrates and correctly expresses its DNA. The spinal cord also releases chemicals that tell the sheath around the spinal cord—called the *Dura matter*—to be flexible and maintain proper tone and tension. That's one of the reasons that you feel better when you exercise, because it facilitates the activation of the mechanoreceptors we discussed in the last section—you could call these "relaxation chemicals"—to help counteract the effects of stress. Under stress, however, the spinal cord's tone changes. It stretches and stiffens, sort of like when you pull hard on a rubber band. This triggers the transmission of nociceptors that shout, "Hey! We're under stress! Kick in the emergency stress response and get us some help!"

If this goes on long enough, your body heads through phase two of stress and approaches phase three. The vertebrae get stuck because of the increased tension in the spinal cord. If the vertebrae get stuck, fluids can no longer stay in the disk, because the joints of the spine are synovial joints and require motion in order to stay hydrated with this important fluid. Without fluid, the disc begins to degenerate. Arthritis creeps in. You may have been told that this happens because you grow older or because it runs in your family. You may be older, and you may have arthritis running in your family—but those two factors are not what is causing your problems.

The real culprit is stress. This degeneration of your discs is a process that can take a long time to manifest. According to some studies, it may take as many as 18 to 20 years of continual or intermittent stress for this process to give you pain symptoms, because most of the pain-receptive nerve fibers are deep within the "communication trunk" of the spinal column. Even though our bodies are slowly "losing life" as communication is hampered, we still think, "I feel good, so I must be healthy. If it's not broken, don't fix it!" Are you beginning to see how dangerous that line of thought is?

That's why my focus will never be your symptoms. My focus is on breaking the stress response that is building up in your body before it causes real damage. I want to restore mobility to your joints so your body can get rest from the stress and begin to adapt and recover. I want to allow motion to come back in the vertebrae, allow fluid to come back in the discs, and open up your nerve pathways once again so that your brain can communicate life to every cell of your body.

Dr. Roger Sperry once said, "Mobility, specifically spinal mobility, is the greatest nutrient to the brain." This is because synovial joint mobility is necessary to send the right chemicals to the brain that will stimulate the cerebellum to counteract the stress response. If we can increase a person's mobility, we can counteract the perpetual stress response they are experiencing without even realizing it. When we are able to do that, we can begin to restore health and the body's ability to stay well.

EVERY CELL OF YOUR BODY SHOULD VIBRATE WITH LIFE

Every single cell in your body is designed to reproduce, recreate, and rejuvenate itself. That's what life does. That's how it works. By giving your body the support it needs through proper nutrition, hydration, and movement, you allow it to produce and reproduce life! Your cells will have the energy to vibrate with health and express themselves as they were designed to do. When this happens, it is possible for you to have a healthy, happy life.

So, while your family history is certainly a factor in your health, it is not inevitable. The other three factors—your external environment, your internal environment, and your lifestyle practices—really determine how your cells express themselves. And while you can't do anything about what you have inherited, you have nearly complete control over your external world, over what you eat, over how much you exercise, and over whether you live your life with purpose or not. In other words, you choose the level of your cellular vibration!

That's the point of Unhealthy Anonymous. We're here to partner with you in your quest for a rich, full life. Let us unite and help each other become good students of our bodies, of nutrition, of how to move effectively, and of caring for others. Let us help each other be better stewards in all the important areas of life, and let us help you facilitate your body's ability to adapt to and recover from stress. Let us help you get healthy and stay healthy with these 12 simple steps that the world's happiest and healthiest people follow every day. It's a simple formula, and we know that it works!

NOTE

1. Eva Bianconi et al., "An estimation of the number of cells in the human body," *Annuls of Human Biology*, vol. 40, no. 6 (November-December 2013), 463-471, http://informahealthcare.com/doi/abs/10.3109/03014460.2013.807878 (accessed September 26, 2014).

Strength

Bernard was right.
The pathogen is nothing;
the terrain is everything.
—attributed to LOUIS PASTEUR

History purports that the words above were spoken by Mr. Pasteur on his deathbed. The story behind them is interesting, and somewhat ironic as Mr. Pasteur was one of the fathers of germ theory and, by extension, the antibiotic age. He theorized that the acute diseases they faced in his day were the result of pathogens, or hostile microbes. His work is the cornerstone of the medical paradigm that has so successfully combated infectious disease that it has nearly doubled life expectancy since the time of the second World War.

The Bernard he would have referred to was Claude Bernard, a colleague of Pasteur's and a physiologist. While Mr. Pasteur was working on experiments to test his theory that disease was caused by pathogens, Mr. Bernard had a slightly different theory. He believed that disease was the result of imbalances of the *milieu intérieur* (the "environment within") or what we call the "interior terrain." If this interior terrain were balanced, then strong, toxic invaders—Pasteur's pathogens—could not make one sick. However, if the internal systems were weak and imbalanced, these microbes could potentially cause sickness. This is why mildly sick people would come to the hospital and often get much sicker during their stay. The pathogens rampant in hospitals before the days of antiseptics would attack their weak systems, and they would grow worse. The doctors who worked in these hospitals, though, who had stronger inner terrains, could go to these same hospitals day after day without getting sick. This idea of a strong and balanced internal environment eventually lead to the idea of *homeostasis* as we understand it today.

Mr. Bernard even pulled a spectacular stunt to prove his theory. To show that the interior terrain was more important than the invasion of pathogens, he drank a glass of water infected with cholera. He was sure his *milieu intérieur* was healthy and strong enough to handle the disease. After hearing about Bernard's continued health in the face of infection from cholera, Pasteur claimed that he had just been lucky. This 150-year-old debate still echoes today. On one side of the debate is the modern medical model for attacking infectious diseases—and on the other side is functional medicine that argues for the strengthening of the "internal terrain" so that the body can fight off disease for itself.

As in all long-standing debates, the truth lies somewhere in the middle. Yes, germs and other hostile micro-organisms can causes sickness, but they will *not* make one sick whose inner terrain is healthy and strong. You most likely know this to be true from your own experience. Sometimes everyone around you is sneezing, coughing, or down with the flu; but miraculously you don't get sick. Other times, if someone sneezes in your direction, you immediately come down with whatever nasty bug is out there. Once you get sick, it seems easier to catch other bugs and harder to get and stay well. This is because the stresses of pain and sickness or the use of antibiotics have altered your inner terrain without your even knowing it.

STRENGTHENING THE "INTERNAL TERRAIN"

If you are following steps one through ten at this point, you are already doing some of the best things you can for your internal health. Getting sufficient rest, eating a detoxifying and nutritional diet, getting regular exercise, restoring spinal mobility, and choosing to live with grace and gratitude are the best practices if you want to improve your internal environment's ability to handle any bugs or viruses that may head your way.

One thing that I would add, however, is to address the internal universe we have in our stomachs and intestinal tracks. And when I say "universe," that is not an exaggeration. It is what is known as the "gut microbiome"—a universe of microbes—the importance of which science is only beginning to recognize. To give you a bit of an overview, the "gut" is the track that runs from your mouth down your esophagus, to your stomach, through your intestines, and out the other end. As odd as this may be to think about, the gut is actually completely "outside" of the body despite the fact that it is inside of us. It is basically one long tube that runs and circles around through us.

Within this tube is a universe of microbes that can either help us or hurt us. To give some perspective, the body has an estimated

37.2 trillion cells. In comparison, researchers believe that the gut biome is made up of approximately 100 trillion microbes, roughly three times the number of cells we have in our body.

Your gut, brain, immune, and hormonal systems are interconnected and impossible to separate or unwind. Recently there has been a flurry of scientific information about how crucial human micro flora (inner terrain) is to genetic expression, immune system, body weight and composition, mental health, memory, and the potentiality of cancer, diabetes, MS, and other chronic diseases.

Many scientists now believe that each of us belongs to a "micro flora type," just as each of us has a blood type. This micro flora type could very well determine your health outcomes more than anything else that has been discovered. The great news is that you can change your gut biome! By adopting the 12 steps outlined in this book, you can change future gene expression by changing your thoughts, words, attitudes, foods, patterns of movement, and ways of relating to the stress in your environment. This is amazingly good news! Even though the scientific study of inherited gut biomes is still in its infancy, we can look forward with anticipation that this will someday be common knowledge—as common as knowing one's blood type.

Having said that, here are some facts which we already know:

- Destroying your gut flora with pharmaceutical drugs, harsh environmental chemicals, and toxic foods is a primary factor in rising disease rates.

- Inflammation (which begins in the gut) may play a critical role in the development of certain cancers.

- Your gut's microbiome signals the release of cytokines. Cytokines are involved in regulating your immune system's response to inflammation and infection.

- Unless we appreciate this relationship between gut biomes and health outcomes, we will not be able to prevent or effectively intervene in many of the chronic diseases that devastate people's lives today.

In order for true healing to occur and to prevent disease from developing, you must continually send your body messages that it is safe and not under attack. The best way to do this is "from your gut." Why from your gut? Because it is there that your "second brain" resides. Did you even know that you have a second brain? We all have a second brain, and it lives in our guts. When you say, "I just had a gut feeling," or "The shock of bad news hit me right in the gut," you are acknowledging that there is more than just food and waste products in there. Embedded in the wall of your gut is your enteric nervous system (ENS). It is responsible for your "gut instincts" that sense danger in your environment. It is the seat of true knowing. When we can't explain something with logic or emotion, we say, "I just know it in my gut." And we are right.

Your two brains communicate all the time, primarily via the nerve that connects them. *Vagus* is Latin for "wandering." The agus nerve "wanders" from your skull down through your chest and abdomen while branching off into other organs like your heart and your stomach. If you eat something that your gut knows you shouldn't eat, it signals the brain to initiate vomiting, diarrhea, heart palpitations, and sweating to get rid of the noxious substance.

A recent article from the Harvard Medical School states the brain and the gut are connected "so intimately that they should be viewed as one system."[1] The gut remembers, as well. If you have ever been violently ill after eating contaminated food, you know that your gut always remembers what food that was, and chances are you don't eat that food again for a very long time!

Imbalances in the gut biome caused by too many antibiotics prescribed in childhood can lead to digestive issues, mood swings, and a condition called "leaky gut," to name a few. Leaky gut is a condition where toxins from our food that would normally be flushed out of our systems penetrate the lining of our digestive systems getting into our blood and wreaking havoc throughout our bodies. These problems have brought about a new health conversation that includes the word *probiotic*. Probiotics are the opposite of antibiotics. They encourage the health and life of good gut flora instead of killing of harmful microbes.

Knowing this helps us understand how gut health affects not only physical health, but also mental health. Not only is much of your serotonin supply (happy hormone) created in your gut, but your gut microbes directly affect your brain—from basic mood swings to depression to conditions like Alzheimer's, autism, and schizophrenia. It is crucially important to build and maintain strong gut flora in the face of constant attacks from:

- Refined sugars
- Genetically modified foods
- Pesticides and herbicides present in all nonorganic farming
- Conventionally raised meats
- Gluten

- Antibiotics

- Chlorinated and fluorinated water

- Pollution

- NSAIDs (over-the-counter pain relievers)

- Stress!

How do we begin to fix a leaky gut? Gut-balancing healthy bacteria and microbes can be found in fermented vegetables like sauerkraut, through yogurt and kefir, and in kombucha (fermented teas). Probiotics that come in capsule form may also prove helpful for this. Needless to say, keep an eye on this relatively new discussion of the gut microbiome and probiotics, and pay attention to the research coming from it. Creating a healthy gut—and healing a leaky gut may be exactly the solution you need for both renewed health, reversal of disease, and long-term, healthy weight loss.

STRENGTHEN MUSCLE AND BONE

Exercising to burn fat is different from exercising to build muscle. The good news is that I have learned both are a matter of working smarter rather than harder. As you will remember from previous chapters, 15 minutes of high intensity interval training (HITT) is the best way to get your heart rate up, activate your muscle-building hormones, and raise your metabolism to burn fat. Muscle building, however, is more about resistance to stress on your bones and muscles, and then giving your body time to rest and recover from that stress. As it does that, it will strengthen your skeleton and build up your muscles. According to the Mayo Clinic:

By stressing your bones, strength training increases bone density and reduces the risk of osteoporosis....

As you gain muscle, your body begins to burn calories more efficiently. The more toned your muscles, the easier it is to control your weight.[2]

Edward R. Laskowski, one of the doctors at the Mayo Clinic, emphasizes that the work of building muscle and strengthening our internal terrain is never completed. According to him, you are either creating muscle or you are creating fat. As he puts it:

If you don't do anything to replace the lean muscle you lose, you'll increase the percentage of fat in your body…. But strength training can help you preserve and enhance your muscle mass—at any age.

Here are some other rather counterintuitive things you should know about building muscle:

- Muscle is built outside of the gym. Muscle is actually built *after* the strain of exercise is over—it is built in recovery, not during exercise. It is part of the body's work to adapt to and recover from the exertion of working out. Thus, if you want to build muscle, you hamper that effort if you never get proper rest, or if you fail to give your body the nutritional building blocks it needs to grow muscle. That generally means plenty of protein and healthy fats.

- An excessive amount of cardio type exercise can hamper your efforts to build muscle. Muscle is built through resistance to weight; cardio burns energy and calories, and may actually shrink muscle mass and reduce strength for a time.

- Working out too long is counterproductive. HGH and testosterone—both necessary for building muscles—peak in the first 30 minutes of exercise and then begin to drop off dramatically after 45 minutes. Cortisol also begins to rise unhealthily after 45 minutes, leading to negative effects like fat production, immune impairment, and cannibalization of muscle.

- It is optimal to limit your repetitions to ten for each set. If you can do 30 repetitions of a certain weight, you are doing more cardio than weight resistance, so you need to lift more weight rather than doing more repetitions. You should be getting tired at ten repetitions. I usually suggest doing three sets of ten repetitions for each exercise, trading off between muscle groups so that you get plenty of rest between each set for the same group of muscles.

- Don't rest too much between exercises. When you are trying to build muscle, you will want to completely fatigue your muscles to encourage them to grow when your body rests, repairs, and rebuilds. You will also want to maximize the release of muscle-building hormones. Considering both of these needs, it is best to limit your rest breaks between repetitions to no more than 90 seconds each.

- Build strength, not just muscle. Work your muscles to build strength in your bones, joints, as well as to maintain muscle. Also, increase flexibility by warming up and cooling down correctly as we talked about in step nine.

- Once again, apply the *connect* principle. Working out with a friend or a group will make the experience more fun, keep you motivated, provide accountability, and even ensure the safety of your workout sessions.

FEED YOUR VISION, STARVE YOUR DISTRACTIONS

It's good to keep in the forefront of our minds why we started this incredible journey in the first place. I'm sure that as you have worked through these steps you have done a good bit of thinking about what you want out of this program, what might trip you up, and what strategies you will use to make these steps part of your regular weekly schedule. At this point, it's time to start pulling those together and focusing on the big picture.

When people start new endeavors like this, too often they make the mistake of focusing on what they don't want rather than on what they do want—or on what they aren't going to do rather than what they are going to do. The negative looms, while the positive fades. Although this is natural, it is not beneficial. In order to make these lifestyle changes, you will need all the positive energy you can muster! If you focus on what you are giving up, or what you are missing out on, then you will be defeated before you begin!

As you begin, take some time to set up cues to remind yourself to feed your vision. One of the things I always suggest is to buy a journal you like and make journaling a new habit. Make the time to write each day about what you want from this program and strategies for making sure that will happen. Keep it with you so that you can record what you eat when you are away from home, or when you eat what you didn't prepare yourself. Use it to record your favorite recipes. Whatever seems important to you for this journey, you can use this journal to keep track of it. Feeling extra energy today? Write it down. Learned a new trick or a new recipe? Write it down! Increased the amount of arm weights you were able to do? Overcame a temptation to eat poorly or not exercise? Write it down and rejoice!

It is also good to keep a list of your goals on the door of your refrigerator—include pictures if you can. Think of the cues that make you want to snack and figure out other routines so that you can change your habits. Plan out your morning and evening rituals so that you will stay the course. Evenings can be the worst, especially if you watch a lot of television and are used to snacking when you do. Change things up by thinking about what you really want to watch and scheduling those times rather than just coming in and looking for something to watch.

If you are like most Americans, you watch a lot more television than you really intend to. Once you get in front of it, it's just too hard to get up and do something else. If you have a DVR, then you can set the TV to record the shows you like and choose when it is most convenient for you to watch them—plus it lets you skip the food commercials featuring mouth-watering, giant pizzas. Think about other things you can do besides watching TV. Too often we forget about fun activities like playing games, helping your kids with homework, reading, or working on a hobby.

Build buffers into your evenings. Plan to have at least an hour of screen-free time before you go to bed. That means no computer, phone, tablet, or television. You will notice that you sleep better as the left and right hemispheres of your brain balance out. Also consider going to bed earlier and getting up earlier to accommodate your exercise, journal writing, prayer and meditation, or other things that can help you set the right tone for your day.

From here on out, you are going to start living intentionally and purposefully doing the things that you have planned. Think about how you want your mornings and evenings to go. Think about how you want your relationships to be, and how you are going to change meals from something you have to do to something you plan to share with others and enjoy. Attitude changes like this will make all the difference in sticking to the 12 steps and making them an integral part of your lifestyle.

BUILDING ON YOUR STRENGTHS

It's easy to focus on the things that you have done wrong in your life. The game of shame and blame is often played alone. This journey may be one step forward and two steps back for you. You may feel guilty when you "cheat" on your program. When this happens, understand the difference between guilt and shame. Guilt is a healthy response to the gap between behaviors that are not up to the standard that we believe we are capable of. We know we can do better, so we feel guilt. Guilt says, "That was a bad action." Shame is destructive. It says, "You are a bad person for doing that behavior." Shame corrodes the piece of us that believes that we can change. So when you are too lazy to exercise, or when you eat too much or allow yourself to exceed your limitations in every way, pick yourself up, dust yourself off, and start all over again. Change is possible, even after messing up!

When these inevitable episodes happen, you may feel as if there is no hope of your ever creating a happier, healthier life. Successful people don't focus on their weaknesses and failure, however;

they focus on their strengths. Professional athletes may not have been the best students when they were in school, but that is not what carried them successfully to the top. Professional chefs don't succeed because they are great accountants; they succeed because they are good cooks. (And they find someone else to keep their books!) People don't succeed by focusing on their weaknesses, but on finding their strengths and maximizing them.

On the 12 steps of this journey, focus on your strengths rather than your weaknesses, on the foods and recipes you like rather than those that someone else says you "should" like, on what you will eat rather than what you are trying to avoid, and on an exercise program that fits with the activities you like rather than those activities that you have never been good at or never enjoyed. When you accentuate the positives in this way, you increase your chances of creating and living the life that you really want.

NOTES

1. "The Gut-brain connection," *Harvard Health Publications* website (March 27, 2012), http://www.health.harvard.edu/healthbeat/the -gut-brain-connection (accessed October 1, 2014).

2. Mayo Clinic Staff, "Strength training: Get stronger, leaner, healthier," Mayo Clinic website (April 24, 2013), http://www .mayoclinic.org/healthy-living/fitness/in-depth/strength-training/ art-20046670 (accessed September 28, 2014).

Generosity

"It is more blessed to give than to receive."
—THE BIBLE

The final of these 12 steps is giving. This step comes last, not because it is the least important, but because it is the crowning glory of all the other steps. If the first 11 steps are the cornerstone, then generosity or giving is the capstone. I cannot emphasize its importance enough. This is not a step that you can check off a checklist; rather, it is an attitude—a way of living that will truly take you to that place of spiritual rest and homeostasis—that place of true contentment that few humans achieve.

Do you know what a capstone is? I didn't until recently when I found out that the process of protecting something built of stone is called *coping*! Isn't the irony of that word amazing? After masons and bricklayers had spent weeks and years of their lives building something, they topped it with a capstone to protect what they had built—and it was called coping. In order to better "cope" with stress, I suggest a conscious, intentional look at your life to see if you are more prone to give, or more prone to hold on to what you have.

The capstone of generosity will allow you to preserve and protect the foundation that has been laid with the previous 11 steps of unhealthy anonymous.

There is a powerful story of unknown origin that simply and beautifully illustrates the essence of generosity. A young boy was reluctantly tagging along with his mother when she was shopping. In and out of stores she went, but not to any interesting stores that had model airplanes or sports equipment. No, she went to perfume stores and antique stores looking for a gift for his grandmother. In one particular store he got bored and began touching the merchandise—an action expressly forbidden by his mother. He shook and rattled jars and vases till he found one that had some treasure inside. He stuck in his hand and felt a coin! Wrapping his chubby little fingers around the coin, he tried to pull it out of the vase but couldn't. Try as he might, he couldn't get his hand out. He was surely in trouble now

Soon his mother found him with a panicky look on his face and tears in his eyes. She also tried to get his hand out without injury, but was unsuccessful. The owner of the store was very upset when she saw that this little boy had his hand stuck in a five thousand dollar antique vase. She tried to remain calm, applying Vaseline to his little hand and to the neck of the expensive antique. No luck. Finally, with much despair the mother agreed to make payments until the vase was paid off if the owner would let her break the vase and save her boy's hand. So she did. After safely cleaning up all the bits of broken porcelain, she held her son's hand in hers. She pried open his little fingers that were sweaty and shaking by this time. Inside his clenched fist she found a copper penny. He hadn't been able to remove his hand from the vase because it was clenched tightly around something that was almost worthless. If he had just unclenched his little fist and opened up his hand, this story would have a happy ending, but he didn't.

How many of us live our lives like this little boy? How many of us are gripping so tightly to things that don't matter that we are losing what is truly valuable? Maybe we are trying to hold on to money, a house, a fancy car, our looks, perhaps an illicit relationship, or an addiction of some sort. Perhaps it is a job that has us imprisoned with "golden handcuffs." We know it is killing us, but we can't leave because the money is too good. Perhaps it is a toxic relationship that we stay in for the same reason. All the while we are giving up our most precious asset—our health. What is the remedy for this? Unclenching our hands and merely letting go in surrender as we realize that if we don't have our health, we don't have anything. If we don't have joy, then what is it all for?

Why do we hang on to so many things that no longer serve us? Fear. We are afraid to let go of them because that would be unfamiliar, and strange, and uncomfortable; and because we have been holding on to them for so long that we can't remember what it feels like to unclench our fists. Here is the secret: When we live life with open hands instead of clenched hands, we learn that there is tremendous abundance in the world—more than enough for everyone on this planet. When we watch the news, we hear about famine, violence, conflict, hunger, scarcity. But there really is enough water and food and air and love for everyone in this world. We don't have a supply problem as humans; we have a distribution problem. I read recently that the amount of money that churchgoers in America spend just on golf each year would solve the world hunger crisis immediately. While I know this to be true, I can't really wrap my mind around why we aren't doing things differently. That is, until I think of that little boy with the penny. He just never thought of unclenching his fist and letting it go.

The secret to happiness is contentment, and the secret to contentment is to actively believe (live like it is true each and every day) that what we have is more than enough. Did you hear that? *More. Than. Enough.* Your mate? Attractive enough. Your house? Big enough. Your kids? Smart enough. Your car? New enough. And on and on. Go through the inventory of your life each day and remind yourself that everything in it is a gift! You really did nothing to deserve being born in good health into one of the richest nations in the world. You did nothing to deserve all the education, the opportunities, the love and joy you have right now. It is enough.

As you begin to live life this way, you will find that giving to others is really not difficult. If someone is hungry, you feed them— because you have enough. If they are thirsty, you give them a drink—because you know you have enough. If they are lonely, you befriend them. If they are grieving, you comfort them. If they are down and out, you help them get up and in. You can always give because you know that we live in a universe that is run by spiritual laws of abundance. Laws that were set in motion before you were ever born. Laws that will continue to rule the world long after you are gone. No matter how much you give to others, you cannot diminish the abundance of the universe. It's that simple.

When you begin to live this way, you will be above the petty annoyances and concerns of life. When you wake up every day knowing that it is a gift you do not deserve, you will look around for other things for which to be grateful. As your gratitude increases, your joy increases. As your joy increases, your cells begin to vibrate at a higher energy level. As your cells vibrate at this higher energy level, they throw off toxins and attract the same level of energy. Good things begin to come into your life. This is the essence of the healthy, happy life—realizing the abundance all around us, being actively grateful for that abundance, sharing that abundance with others while we ourselves are being blessed with contentment, joy, and peace. I wish this for you, today and every day.

PLUGGING IN TO YOUR LOCAL UA COMMUNITY

The center of Unhealthy Anonymous is the communities formed in your local health center, recreation center, community hall, place of worship, or school. It is a place first and foremost to connect with like-minded persons who have similar health goals, and second, to continue the conversation we have started in this book. While we were able to discuss overarching principles, you will still need a place to gather and get more details about eating real food, healing your body, and returning all systems to a place of homeostasis and rest.

Each meeting will have new information to educate you on the benefits of good nutrition, exercise, and other lifestyle choices, as well as helpful tips and inside information about how to make a habitual lifestyle of healthy choices. They will also have regular segments like "Shopping with the Doc" that will educate you and empower you in practical ways.

If you bought this book online or somewhere other than a UA group, and don't know of one in your area, please go to www.unhealthyanonymous.com to see if you can find one, or to get information on how to start one in your area.

IF YOU REALLY WANT TO LEARN SOMETHING, TEACH IT

Another way to practice giving is to share this information with others. One reason to do this is that if you really want to understand it, the best way to do that is to explain it to someone else. The Roman philosopher Seneca expressed this idea thousands of years ago when he said, "While we teach, we learn." Nothing proves how well you understand a concept as being able to help someone else understand it. Find someone who needs this information, and share it with him. You might just save his life!

This sharing is one of the key pillars of Unhealthy Anonymous: We are a community of people learning together and offering support and accountability for this new lifestyle. The concepts we have touched on in this book are a mere overview—we have set the foundation, but the real work of building the rest of the house is up to you. Health is a rapidly evolving field. We are learning new things every day, and as we do, it will change the entire conversation about how we deal with stress as well as how we get and stay healthy. Having a place to get the latest, most up-to-date information from people you trust is a powerful asset in the quest for health.

After all, there is so much conflicting information out there. Take, for example, some of the myths we have dealt with throughout this book:

Myth: "Losing weight makes you healthy."

Actually, getting healthy will allow you to maintain a healthy weight

Myth: "Losing weight is a matter of calories in and calories out."

Many doctors still tell their patients today that losing weight is a simple formula: eat fewer calories + burn more calories = weight loss. But we know now that when your body is under stress, your cortisol levels are elevated, causing you to accumulate fat around your vital organs.

Myth: "All calories are the same."

Even a grade school student can tell you that 1,000 calories of soda in a Big Gulp is not the same as 1,000 calories of broccoli. The issue is not the calories, but the fiber and micronutrient contents in the food.

Myth: "You get fat from eating fat."

As we have learned, not all fats are alike. The fats in grain-fed beef are different from the fats in lean, grass- or green-fed beef. The fats in processed foods are different from the fats in an avocado or wild-caught fish. Good fats turn off your hunger and create satisfaction that lasts for hours.

Myth: "The _____ diet is the latest, greatest, and only one you will ever need."

God made an abundance of food choices for us, and no one program of eating is going to be right for everyone. We all have different body types, different cultural backgrounds, different taste buds, and different demands on our time. That's why a program of eating based on sound nutrition with a myriad of choices is optimal.

"Heart disease is caused by eating beef."

Heart disease and arterial plaque are caused by overconsumption of grains and sugars as well as breathing toxic air.

Myth: "Breakfast is the most important meal of the day."

Usually the ones saying that are the people selling breakfast foods. And then they surround their sugary cereals with a bunch of other foods and tell you that it's a balanced breakfast. Bah! Intermittent fasting is a great way to give all your cells the rest they need.

There are other myths of course, and I encourage you to research these myths and confront them with the truth. This isn't so you can be a know-it-all, but so you can join in the discussions where you will inevitably hear about what is good for you and what isn't. Be an advocate for these truths. Remember, our goal isn't to be right; our goal is to help people get healthy so that they don't experience what 80 percent of Americans are experiencing today—lives characterized by chronic disease and discomfort. Education is a lifelong process. Keep learning, growing, and teaching others. This is the best way to stay young and remain relevant!

CHANGED LIVES WILL CHANGE THE WORLD

This is not a political movement or a radical ideological revolution. This is a movement of friends and neighbors coming together to make a difference in our own lives and the lives of the generations that will follow us. When the bubonic plague swept through Europe, it killed roughly a third of the population. It changed the world and the way people looked at sickness and disease. Today we have a plague of lifestyle diseases that are crippling and killing millions. These preventable diseases overload our healthcare system, cost us trillions of dollars a year, and feed the businesses whose principals are content to trade our nation's health for the bottom line on their income statements and shareholder profits. This needs to change, and it needs to change now.

The good news is that, although it may take years to change our country's culture, it will only take a couple of weeks to change the culture of your own household. You will be surprised at how quickly switching to a real food diet and getting a little exercise every day will change the way you feel, change how food tastes to you, and eventually transform the way you look and feel.

REVERSING THE PANDEMIC

I believe we are on the forefront of a new health revolution that will point people back to real foods and create a new paradigm of health that focuses on health rather than sickness. Functional medicine is growing in popularity and influence. Current research shows us that our best ally against diseases of all kinds is a healthy body—not pharmaceuticals; not extreme surgeries; not the latest, greatest antidepressant; not a new potent supplement or extreme diet or workout fad. It all starts with what Hippocrates and others knew thousands of years ago:

> The natural healing force within each of us is the greatest force in getting well. And if we could give every individual the right amount of nourishment and exercise, not too little and not too much, we would have found the safest way to health.

Change your life. Change the future health of your children. Make sure you will be around to play with your great-grandchildren. Spread the word. More people need to join this movement. It is time to change our nation's health for the better. There are missions to be filled, great deeds to be done, discoveries to be made, products to be invented, lives to be changed; but you won't be around to be an active part of all this if you are sick or dead. It's time to grab hold of the 12 steps of Unhealthy Anonymous and spread the word about how to live happy and healthy lives. Let's go after this great adventure together!

About the Author

DR. PETE SULACK is the founder of Unhealthy Anonymous, an organization that helps individuals, corporations and non-profits understand and manage the immense effects of stress. Founder and majority owner of one of the largest Chiropractic clinics in North America, he has served over 1 million patients over the last 12 years, validating his unique approach to health and wellness. Dr. Pete actively treats patients traveling from around the world seeking his services. His studies on the effects of stress, coupled with testimonials from patients and attention in medical communities have garnered him the title of America's Leading Stress Expert. He is a highly sought-after teacher, lecturer and author of several books.

DESTINY IMAGE BOOKS BY DR. PETE SULACK

The Joseph Blessing

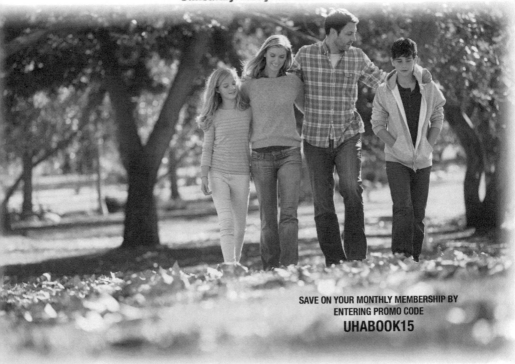

Dr. Pete Sulack
AMERICA'S LEADING STRESS EXPERT

**PRIVATE ACCESS
24/7 - 365**

UNHEALTHYANONYMOUS.COM

❤📖 LOVE to READ?

Get FREE eBooks,
Deep Discounts and New Release Updates!

Sign up now.
destinyimage.com/freebooks

📚 SHARE this BOOK!

Don't let the impact of this book end with you!

Get a discount
when you order

3 or MORE BOOKS.
CALL 1-888-987-7033

🎤 AUTHOR INTERVIEWS

Exclusive interviews with your favorite authors!

Tune in today.
voiceofdestiny.net

 Destiny Image is a division of Nori Media Group.